GOOD
FOOD
FOR
BAD
STOMACHS

GOOD

FOOD

for

BAD

STOMACHS

Henry D. Janowitz, M.D.

New York   Oxford
OXFORD UNIVERSITY PRESS
1997

Oxford University Press

Oxford   New York
Athens   Auckland   Bangkok   Bogotá   Bombay
Buenos Aires   Calcutta   Cape Town   Dar es Salaam
Delhi   Florence   Hong Kong   Istanbul   Karachi
Kuala Lumpur   Madras   Madrid   Melbourne
Mexico City   Nairobi   Paris   Singapore
Taipei   Tokyo   Toronto

and associated companies in
Berlin   Ibadan

Copyright © 1997 by Henry D. Janowitz

Published by Oxford University Press, Inc.
198 Madison Avenue, New York, New York 10016

Oxford is a registered trademark of Oxford University Press

The author gratefully acknowledges Consumer Reports for information
included in Table 2; and Celiac Sprue Association, U.S.A., Inc.
for information included in Table 8.

Library of Congress Cataloging-in-Publication Data
Janowitz, Henry D.
Good food for bad stomachs /
Henry D. Janowitz.
p.   cm.   Includes index.
ISBN 0–19–508792–5
1. Gastrointestinal system—Diseases—Diet therapy.
2. Indigestion—Popular works.
I. Title.
RC816.J36   1997   616.3'30654—dc20   96–9409

1 3 5 7 9 8 6 4 2

Printed in the United States of America
on acid-free paper

*This book is dedicated to
the many patients
whose persistent questions
stimulated it.*

ACKNOWLEDGMENTS

✳ ✳ ✳

Although I had the title of this book in mind for a long time, that I did write it is due to the persistent and unfailing support given me by my editor at Oxford, Joan Bossert, the editors of *Consumer Reports*, and my agent, Ms. Ruth Wrechner. They deserve and have my thanks. My wife, Adeline R. Tintner, gave it a layperson's interested and thorough review. Its faults, I need hardly add, are my own.

CONTENTS

✳ ✳ ✳

TABLES

✱ ✱ ✱

I

GOOD FOOD FOR GOOD STOMACHS

1

* * *

WHAT THIS BOOK
IS ABOUT

To begin with, let me tell you what this book is *not* about. It is not a diet book: it won't tell you how to lose weight, reduce your blood's bad cholesterol levels, and rev up the "good" cholesterol without counting calories, while you eat all and everything you want. It is not about food as the elixir of lost youth. It is not about eating as a way to improve your immune system.

What then is this book about?

I will present in an orderly way what we know about the role of our eating habits in preventing, causing, and treating the many disorders that plague our gastrointestinal tract and its associated digestive glands—the liver, gallbladder, and pancreas. Our aim is to separate what is known in this complicated and interesting field from what is not known about those special factors that influence our digestive health. If possible, this book should help in sifting the facts from the myths. There are few topics about which we see so many conflicting ideas as this one of food and digestion. There are indeed few areas in medicine so loaded with emotion and assumptions as diet.

As the starting point for the book, the preliminary chapters tentatively approach the question, "Is there such a thing as an ideal diet?" We need to look at what our nutritional requirements are first. We need to know what we require daily in the way of calories, carbohydrates, proteins, and fat, as well as the obligatory vitamins and trace elements. We need to know something about the amount of fiber and calcium our diet ought to contain, but we must bear in mind that the amounts published by various scientific bodies also reflect compromises between different varying and vocal advocates and are often changed as more nutritional information is available. There are scientific fads, just as there are other fads. There are perpetual changes centering around such "trendy" subjects as animal versus non-animal fat, or saturated versus unsaturated fatty acids. Margarine was okay until a short time ago; now we are to worry about *cis* and *trans* forms. I do not think I am giving away my subject prematurely when I say that we do not know what the "ideal diet" should be; we can, however, formulate the elements of a realistic, reasonable diet.

That being the case, I devote a chapter to the concept of an ideal diet and offer the current consensus of those working in the field on what constitutes a "healthy" diet. The old proverb still holds that we are what we eat, *Mann ist was Mann esst*, and we all seem to agree with Walter de la Mare's little rhyme:

> *It's a very odd thing—*
> *As odd as it can be—*
> *That whatever Miss T eats*
> *Turns into Miss T.*

There is one fact that always strikes me as important as well as interesting. The human digestive system evolved over millions of years (between 100 and 50 million years), adapting to the existing environment of our hunting and food-gathering primitive ancestors. While there has probably been no evidence of any evolutionary changes in the human digestive tract in recorded time (10 million years), the sustaining nutritional environment has changed radically, perhaps never more so than in the last one hundred years. Can this be the source of any of our current digestive problems? We might get some insight into this question by speculating about what the human prehistoric diet was or may have been that has changed so radically.

Other portions of the book are devoted to intestinal gas, constipation, diarrhea, the effect of aging, the effects of food on drug absorption, and the several effects of drugs on food absorption.

But the bulk of this book looks at the kinds of disorders that may and do occur from one end of the digestive tract to the other, and our attempts to define, if possible, the role of diet in preventing, causing, or treating these disorders. How can we treat these digestive diseases and still maintain a healthy intake of food? What compromises can be made with the limitations that the disease imposes on our optimal nutritional goals, and how do we compensate for these limiting factors? If we don't eat what we should, what risks do we run, and how do we overcome them?

We also look at esophagitis and swallowing disorders, inflammation and ulcers of the stomach and duodenum (especially peptic ulcer and gastritis), gallstones, pancreatitis, acute and chronic liver disease, as well as traveler's diarrhea, constipation, inflammation and defects of the small intestine, disorders such as sprue, along with the role of diet in colonic polyps and colon rectal cancer.

I try to approach the vexatious problem of food intolerances, food allergies, and food reactions in an effort to separate the known from the unknown, realizing that we still act and eat as though we don't have all the answers. I pay special attention to the group of inflammatory bowel diseases, which includes ulcerative colitis and Crohn's disease, as well as the ubiquitous irritable bowel syndrome. I also spend a considerable amount of time discussing two areas in which diet plays an important part of therapy—one is the problem presented by patients with gluten enteropathy, celiac disease, or sprue, as it is called, where the need for a gluten-free diet is essential; the other problem involves oxalate metabolism and the formation of kidney oxalate stones, in disorders of the small intestine. In both of these, diet may play a central role.

2

✻ ✻ ✻

IS THERE AN
IDEAL DIET?

America is health conscious. Everyone, or so it seems, is attempting to follow a physical fitness program; everyone is "working out"; everyone is eating a special diet and trying to lose weight.

We all want to eat a healthy diet. Yet we don't really know whether there is an ideal diet we all should strive to attain. The problem is not lack of information. There is almost too much information. The daily newspapers, the radio and T.V. health programs, the weekly and monthly magazines not only are asking us if we are eating correctly, but advising us in detail what to eat and what to avoid.

Authoritative institutions are waving their arms to get our attention. The U.S. Department of Agriculture publishes and distributes its attractive folder of the "Food Guide Pyramid—Beyond the Basic 4" (Figure 1). The American Heart Association also announces and revises its recommendations in an effort to avoid heart disease. And in my supermarket, the plastic shopping bags carry a message from the National Cancer Institute: "Nature's Fast Food—Eat Five Fruits and Vegetables a Day," boldly announcing in italics that "35 percent of all cancer deaths can be attributed to the typical American diet which is too high in fat and too low in fiber"—urging us that "eating more fruit and vegetables could be the most important lifestyle change you ever make."

All the experts agree that our natural eating and drinking habits are involved in at least six of the ten leading causes of death—heart disease, cancer, stroke, diabetes, hardening of the arteries (atherosclerosis), chronic liver disease, and cirrhosis of the liver, and are probably closely related to osteoporosis and diverticulosis. All the experts agree that we should follow a diet that contains a large portion of complex carbohydrates (vegetables, fruits, and grains) and is high in fiber and low in fats (avoiding saturated fats and cholesterol). Indeed, in a recent survey conducted by *Consumer Reports*, the experts do take their own advice seriously and follow their own recommendations. The problem is not the generalities but translating these simple generalities into the everyday diet.

Eating for Health

Weight Control and Caloric Intake

I have already pointed out that this book is not a weight reduction primer. There is no miracle road to weight loss. Calories do count and you can't eat all you want, of what you enjoy, and still lose weight. But certain points should be stressed at this junction in our discussion.

There is no doubt that being overweight increases the chance of getting high blood pressure and diabetes, but these disorders improve, and in some individuals quite dramatically, when you lose 10 percent of your weight or even less. So it is worthwhile watching your diet, even if you aren't interested in

Table 1. Suggested Weights for Adults

Height[a]	Weight in Pounds[b]	
	19 to 34 years	35 years and older
5'0"	97–128	108–138
5'1"	101–132	111–143
5'2"	104–137	115–148
5'3"	107–141	119–152
5'4"	111–146	122–157
5'5"	114–150	126–162
5'6"	118–155	130–167
5'7"	121–160	134–172
5'8"	125–164	138–178
5'9"	129–169	142–183
5'10"	132–174	146–188
5'11'	136–179	151–194
6'0"	140–184	155–199
6'1"	144–189	159–205
6'2"	148–195	164–210
6'3"	152–200	168–216
6'4"	156–205	173–222
6'5"	160–211	177–228
6'6"	164–216	182–234

Note: The higher weights in the ranges generally apply to men, who tend to have more muscle and bone; the lower weights more often apply to women, who have less muscle and bone.

[a] Without shoes
[b] Without clothes

Source: Dietary Guidelines for Americans, published by the U.S. Department of Agriculture and the Department of Health and Human Services.

reaching the ideal weight the insurance company tables tell you to aim for.

There are a number of ideal weight tables prepared and available from life insurance actuarial studies, though many in this field prefer to use the Dietary Guidelines for Americans that furnish the range for men and women in age groups (19 to 34 years, and 35 years and older; see Table 1).

Deviating a few pounds from these ranges does not really pose a problem. It is being grossly overweight (20 percent over the guidelines) that does. But losing a substantial amount of weight is never easy and requires additional outputs of energy—which means regular exercise. It appears that the added weight, which is essentially fat around the waist, is of greater risk to your health than weight that is around the hips and thighs. So if your waist is larger than your hips or thigh measurements, you should consider some weight reduction. A general prescription of a diet high in carbohydrates, low in fat, and high in fiber would suit these individuals very well. But a major reduction in weight (20 percent or more) is always difficult and maintaining that lower weight by any method is still more difficult. Relapses occur all too frequently and invariably in some individuals.

What is important to keep in mind is that repeated weight loss followed by repeated regains may be even worse than not losing weight at all. This "yo-yo" movement has been shown to have a bad effect, especially for the cardiovascular system of the individual, although this too has been recently challenged.

Yet, despite their best efforts, some people may be genetically predisposed to particular metabolic patterns that may prevent permanent weight loss. For these individuals, following a low-fat, high-fiber, high-carbohydrate diet may be the best and wisest thing they can do. If you are among these people, then establishing good dietary habits should be your main concern rather than frantic worrying about what your weight scale tells you.

Whatever Happened to the Food Pyramid?

I have already mentioned the Food Guide Pyramid program published by the U.S. Department of Agriculture, which was based on the recommendations of a panel of distinguished nutritionists. The pyramid (Figure 1) is divided into five groups and suggests the following daily servings:

- 6 to 11 servings of cereals, bread, rice, and pasta
- 3 to 5 servings of vegetables

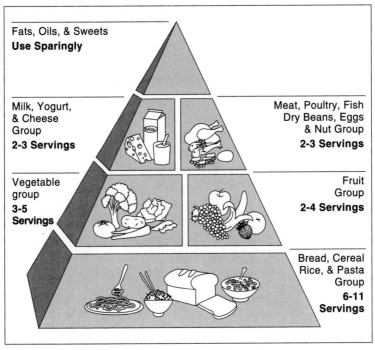

Figure 1. The Food Pyramid

- 2 to 3 servings of low-fat milk products—milk, cheese, or yogurt
- 2 to 4 servings of fruit
- 2 to 3 servings of meat, poultry, fish, dried beans, eggs, or nuts

  Fats, oils, and sweets are to be used sparingly.
  What counts as a serving?

- One slice of bread, one ounce of ready-to-eat cereal, a half-cup of cooked cereal, rice, or pasta
- A cup of green leafy vegetables, a half-cup of other vegetables cooked or chopped, three-quarters of a cup of vegetable juice
- One cup of milk or yogurt, 1 ½ ounces of natural cheese
- One medium-sized apple, banana, or orange, one of chopped, canned, or cooked fruit, three-quarters of a cup of fruit juice

- Two to three ounces of lean cooked meat, poultry, or fish, a half-cup of dried beans, or one egg; two tablespoons of peanut butter counts as one ounce of lean meat

We could attempt to apply the Food Guide Pyramid in actual dietary use by following the suggestions of *Consumer Reports* (October 1992) presented in Table 2.

The pyramid suggests we eat more fruits and vegetables and less sweets, cheese, fried foods, and rich desserts. Now that we have gotten that fixed in our minds and, more important, served on our plates, along comes a new pyramid—the *Mediterranean pyramid*—with equally good credentials. The World Health Organization, the Collaboratory Center for Nutrition of the Harvard School of Public Health, and Oldways Preservation and Exchange Trust, a Boston group which seeks to preserve traditions in food, all endorse this new pyramid. But what is new here that we can apply to our diets?

This pyramid is based on diets eaten in certain parts of the Mediterranean world that seem to be free of some forms of chronic disease. In contrast to the U.S. Department of Agriculture pyramid, the Mediterranean diet recommends no more than 12 ounces of meat a month, suggests the very liberal use of olive oil, and allows more than 35 percent of the total calories of the diet to come from fat, as compared with the U.S. Agricultural level of 25 percent of total calories from fat. It also suggests wine in moderation—one to two glasses per day for men, one glass per day for women.

The core of the diet relies on bread, pasta, and rice along with couscous, bulgur, and other grains, vegetables, beans, and olive oil on everything. Fish could be eaten a few times a week, poultry less often, and red meat a few times a month.

Now that we have fairly adopted and adapted to the U.S. pyramid, I am reluctant to advise the Mediterranean pyramid. I remind readers of the flurry of interest in drinking red wine which is said to protect the French when they consume as much fatty goose liver as they wish without getting into trouble with

Table 2. Suggested Do's and Don'ts for Food Choices

Choose Often	Choose Sometimes	Choose Rarely (or in very small amounts)
Milk, Yogurt, and Cheese Group: 2 to 3 Servings		
Skim and 1% low-fat milk	2% low-fat milk	Whole milk
Buttermilk made with skim or 1% low-fat milk	Buttermilk made with 2% low-fat milk	
Yogurt made with skim or 1% low-fat milk	Yogurt made with 2% low-fat milk	Yogurt made with whole milk
	Hot cocoa or chocolate milk from skim or 1% milk	Hot cocoa or chocolate milk from 2% milk
	Puddings made with skim or 1% milk	Puddings made with 2% or whole milk
1% low-fat or dry-curd cottage cheese	2% cottage cheese	Creamed or regular (4% fat) cottage cheese
Cheeses with 2 or fewer grams of fat per ounce	Cheeses with 3 to 5 grams of fat per ounce	Cheeses with more than 5 grams of fat per ounce
Frozen dairy desserts with 2 grams of fat or less per item or per ½-cup serving	Frozen dairy desserts with 3 to 5 grams of fat per item or per ½-cup serving	Ice cream and frozen dairy desserts with more than 5 grams of fat per item or per ½-cup serving

(continued)

Table 2. Suggested Do's and Don'ts for Food Choices (continued)

Choose Often	Choose Sometimes	Choose Rarely (or in very small amounts)
Meat, Poultry, Fish, Dry Beans, Eggs, and Nuts Group: 2 to 3 Servings		
Beef: Eye of round, top round	Beef: Tip or bottom round, sirloin, chuck arm, pot roast, top loin, tenderloin, flank, T-Bone steak	Beef: Porterhouse steak, brisket, chuck blade roast, rib-eye, ribs, short ribs, ground beef (even "lean" or "extra lean"), liver, corned beef, pastrami, bologna, salami, frankfurters
Veal: All cuts except loin, rib, and ground	Veal: Loin, rib chop, ground	
Pork: Tenderloin	Pork: Sirloin chop, top or center loin chop, rib chop, ham, Canadian bacon	Pork: Blade steak, bacon, pepperoni, sausage, frankfurters, bologna, salami
Lamb: Foreshank	Lamb: Shank half, leg, sirloin half, loin chop	Lamb: Rib chop, arm, blade, shoulder, ground lamb
Chicken breast without skin; turkey breast or leg; turkey wing without skin; ground turkey without skin	Chicken breast with skin; chicken leg, thigh, or wing without skin; turkey wing with skin	Chicken leg, thigh, or wing with skin; chicken liver; ground turkey with skin; duck and goose; poultry frankfurters
Poultry cold cuts with up to 1 gram of fat per ounce	Poultry cold cuts with 2 grams of fat per ounce	Poultry cold cuts, 3 or more grams of fat per ounce

Choose Often	Choose Sometimes	Choose Rarely (or in very small amounts)
All fresh fish and shellfish	Smoked fish	
Canned fish, water-packed, drained	Canned fish, oil-packed, drained	
All dried beans, peas, and lentils	Soybeans, tofu	Nuts, peanuts, and other nut butters
Egg whites	Egg substitutes	Whole eggs or yolks
Vegetable Group: 3 to 5 Servings		
Fresh vegetables or frozen vegetables without sauce	Canned vegetables, vegetable juices	Frozen vegetables in sauce
Fruit Group: 2 to 4 Servings		
All fresh fruit (except avocado and olives)	Dried fruit, fruit juices	Avocado, olives
Unsweetened applesauce	Canned fruit in its own juice	Canned fruit in heavy syrup Sweetened applesauce
Bread, Cereal, Rice, and Pasta Group: 6 to 11 Servings		
Bread, bagels, pita	Egg breads, such as challah and egg bagels; French toast; pancakes; waffles	Bread stuffing; croissants

(continued)

Table 2. Suggested Do's and Don'ts for Food Choices (continued)

Choose Often	Choose Sometimes	Choose Rarely (or in very small amounts)
Muffins, biscuits, or rolls with 2 or fewer grams of fat (e.g., English muffins, hamburger buns)	Muffins, biscuits, and rolls with 3 to 4 grams of fat each	Muffins, biscuits, and rolls with more than 4 grams of fat each
Unbuttered air-popped popcorn, pretzels, rice cakes, bread sticks		Oil-popped and/or buttered popcorn
Corn tortillas	Flour tortillas	
Crackers with 1 gram or less of fat per ½ ounce (e.g., melba toast, matzoh, flatbread, saltines)	Crackers with 2 grams of fat per ½ ounce, such as graham crackers	Crackers with 3 or more grams of fat per ½ ounce, such as Ritz crackers
Cold cereals with 2 or fewer grams of fat and 6 or fewer grams of sugar per serving (e.g., Cheerios, corn flakes, shredded wheat, Grape Nuts)	Cold cereals high in sugar or fat (e.g., granola)	
Hot cereals		
Rice, barley, bulgur wheat, couscous, kasha, quinoa		
Pasta	Egg noodles	

Source: Adapted from Gail A. Levey, M.S., R.D., spokesperson, American Dietetic Association.

elevated blood cholesterol levels. But do we really know the reason for the lower incidence of cardiac disease among the French compared with Americans?

One final ironic note. The Mediterranean diet was eaten in many regions of the Mediterranean until some time in the 1960s, but as some regions became more affluent, their diets also became richer in fat. So while they haven't caught up to the average American intake of fat, they are well on their way.

The Diet of Our Ancestors

Having for a long time considered the possibility of discrepancies between the diet adapted by the gastrointestinal tract of one hundred million years ago, in the Paleolithic Age, and the current Western world's diet transformed especially in the last one to two hundred years, I obviously thought it important to try to find out what scientists, especially anthropologists, could tell us about the Paleolithic diet of the hunters and gatherers of food, our former ancestors.

My task was simplified by the discovery of the studies of S. Boyd Eaton, M.D., Marjorie Shostik, and Melvin Konner, Ph.D., M.D. of Emory University School of Medicine who put their discoveries together in a volume called *The Paleolithic Prescription* (New York: Harper & Row, 1988). For those interested in pursuing this further, I highly recommend this book.

They contrasted the late Paleolithic diet with the contemporary American diet, at the time of their writing, by updating a table that they had published in the *New England Journal of Medicine* 312(5): 283–289 (1985).

Compared to our current American diet, our Paleolithic ancestors ate three times as much protein and half the fat we do. They ate meat, but it was much less fatty than our current animal sources of meat being lean game. Thus the fat they did eat was more polyunsaturated than saturated. They ate very little refined carbohydrates and no finely ground flour. They consumed twice as much calcium as we do. They consumed five to ten times more nonnutrient fiber—a substantial difference. And they didn't smoke or drink alcohol.

It is quite clear from this abbreviated account that the current recommendations from our official authorities are in general fairly close to the diet of our ancestors of forty thousand years ago.

	Late Paleolithic Diet	Contemporary American Diet
Source of Total Daily Dietary Energy (%)		
Protein	33	12
Carbohydrates	46	46
Fat	21	42
Alcohol	0	7–10
Cholesterol (mg)	520	300–500
Sodium (mg)	690	2300–6900
Calcium (mg)	1500–2000	740
Ascorbic acid (mg)	440	90
Fiber (grams)	100–150	20

Preparation of Food: Raw versus Cooked

So far I have spent little time on the question of what effect the preparation of food has on its nutritional value. The chemical components of protein, fat, and carbohydrates are little affected by the mode of cooking, but their availability for the body, especially vegetable nutrients, is affected by the cooking process.

All cooks know that overcooking and overboiling vegetables destroys much of their vitamin content, but eating vegetables raw may not be the best way either. The problem with raw or hard vegetables, especially those rich in fiber like carrots or broccoli, is that these nutrients are often bound into a matrix of fiber in the plants. This does not hold true for soft foods of lower fiber content like peaches and cantaloupe, which are nutritionally better eaten raw. Heating hard vegetables gently breaks down the fiber and allows the individual to absorb much more of the vegetable's nutrients. Only vitamin C is found in high concentrations in raw vegetables; hence the loss of vitamin C is offset by the gain in absorption. Some cooking also makes starch more digestible. Only 30 percent of potato starch is digested when eaten raw compared with 98 percent when cooked. Vegetables such as cauliflower and broccoli contain large amounts of starch that profit from heating.

So the best way to prepare these vegetables is to heat them long enough to loosen up the fibrous matrix and use as little water as possible. Steaming does not damage vitamins, but vegetables should be heated until they are just al dente, tender but still firm. Vitamin C is retained if asparagus, broccoli, cauliflower, and brussels sprouts are steamed in this way.

3

* * *

GUIDELINES FOR
GOOD HEALTH:
THE DO'S AND DON'TS

Fat

According to the "Dietary Guidelines for Americans"—a
joint venture of the U.S. Department of Agriculture, the
Department of Health and Human Services, and the American
Heart Association—our total dietary fat intake should not exceed 30 percent of our daily calories. This translates into 90
grams for active men and teenage boys (where the daily intake
of calories is 2800 calories), 70 grams for children, active
women, and most men (in a 2200-calories-per-day diet), and 50
grams for many women and older adults (in a 1600-calories-
per-day diet). These limits on total fat are directed at the prevention of obesity, some cancers, and especially coronary heart
disease (heart attack).

All interested in these problems urge us to reduce the percentage of saturated fat we eat to 7 percent, or even less.

Types of Fat

Having raised the question of fats in our diet, we need to distinguish their different types.

Saturated Fats All fats are composed of fatty acids, linked in chains and attached to glycerol. In the saturated fats, also called *hydrogenated* fats, a hydrogen atom replaces a double bond between carbon atoms. These fats are solid or hard at room temperature and are found in animal and milk fat. Palm and coconut oil are also saturated fats, but are liquid at room temperature. These saturated dietary fats raise blood cholesterol even more than dietary cholesterol, since the liver converts them into cholesterol.

Unsaturated Fats These are fats similar to those found in olive and peanut oils and are liquid at room temperature and remain soft when refrigerated. Most do not raise serum cholesterol and therefore are to be preferred to saturated fats for people with high serum cholesterol levels. When a hydrogen atom is missing between two adjacent carbon atoms, a stable double bond forms between the adjacent carbons. Fatty acids with one double bond are called *monounsaturated*, and those with two or more double bonds are called *polyunsaturated*. Both are to be preferred to saturated fats.

Cholesterol Cholesterol itself deserves a separate discussion. Most authorities would limit our daily cholesterol intake to 300 milligrams a day, the equivalent of one egg yolk.

In thinking about the contents of this book, I had not expected or intended to devote much text to the cholesterol problem in relation to healthy individuals, but the public is deluged with the accumulating research that has a confusing effect on our recommendations.

While findings on the role of elevated blood cholesterol, the protective role of the high-density lipoproteins (HDLs), and the bad effects of the low-density lipoproteins (LDLs) seem secure enough, some disquieting reports have raised the question whether, in addition to a very high level of cholesterol, a very low level may not also have a down side. Although the death rate is clearly increased with high blood cholesterol values (240 or more milligrams per 100 milliliters), it would appear from some recent studies that very low levels (below 160) increase the risk of intracranial bleeding, liver cancer, noncancerous lung disease, and even suicide or alcoholism! No one knows how to interpret these findings, but my simpleminded philosophy would be to stay with what you are eating if your cholesterol is in the normal range and reduce your cholesterol intake if you are in the elevated range. If you have a very low cholesterol level, I don't have any advice, except to be sure your very low level does not represent an underlying disease, or a poor diet.

What about Nuts? We all enjoy eating walnuts but suffer from the notion that this food family, nuts, is full of fat and of little nutritive value. A recent study has shown that eating walnuts can lower the body's blood cholesterol level. The full explanation for this is not known, but in walnuts 70 percent of the fat is *polyunsaturated*, the "good" as opposed to the "bad" fat. Walnuts also contain large amounts of linolenic and omega-3 fatty acids believed to be essential for our metabolism and which have been shown to reduce blood cholesterol. A quarter of a cup of walnuts has 130 calories, no cholesterol, 4 grams of protein, and a large dose of linolenic acid.

Are There Any Good Fats?

Is margarine a harmful food?

For many years nutritionists have scolded us for eating saturated fat, and food manufacturers have switched from palm or coconut oil and lard to partial hydrogenated vegetable oils made from soybean or corn oil (polyunsaturates). Now they tell us that these oils found in margarine, vegetable shortening, and products such as cookies and doughnuts contain substances that can also cause heart disease.

The suspected ingredient, *trans fatty acid*, is produced when vegetable oils, containing the *cis* form of fatty acids, are converted into margarine or shortening, which is solid or semisolid at room temperature. These *trans* fatty acids, like the saturated fats, tend to raise the harmful elements in blood cholesterol and reduce the high-density lipoproteins (the HDLs) that are so helpful. The bottom line for us is to eat less fat, and we will thus be eating less *trans* fatty acids.

Researchers calculate that Americans eat anywhere from 11 to 28 grams of *trans* fat a day, which is as much as 20 percent of the daily fat intake. They are found in cookies, pastries, cakes, doughnuts, french fries, potato chips, but also in frozen fish sticks, ready-made frostings, and chicken nuggets. A whopping 10 grams can be found in fast-food chicken and fish, and 8 grams is typical in a large portion of french fries cooked or hashed in hydrogenated vegetables oils. Tub margarine is lower in *trans* fat than stick margarine. Lower still are soft margarines or liquid margarines in squeeze bottles; the softer the better.

Olive oil and canola oil are the best choices for cooking. They contain almost no fats other than the oil.

What about Fish Oil?

A good deal of nutritional interest these days centers around fish oil and fish oil supplements for the diet. These fish oils, known as *omega-3 fatty acids*, contain two such oils—eicosapentaenoic acid and desahexaenoic acid. They are prominently displayed in health food windows and enjoy tremendous sales in these stores.

The entire field was given a great start by the observation that Greenland Eskimos with a diet rich in marine oils have fewer heart attacks and strokes caused by abnormal clots than their countrymen in Denmark. It was soon learned that the fish they consumed so avidly contain oils that lower the fat of the blood, the *triglycerides*. They also have a powerful anticlotting effect.

Especially intriguing was the hope that these substances would be helpful in autoimmune diseases, such as rheumatoid arthritis. And some improvement in joint stiffness and distress has been shown in patients with rheumatoid arthritis when they take fish oil supplements. These oils also seem to help chronic migraine sufferers who have not responded to conventional therapy, and modest improvement has been shown in some patients with ulcerative colitis. Smokers with pulmonary diseases, such as chronic bronchitis or emphysema, seem to be helped by these fish oil supplements as well.

But the wholesale use of fish oil supplements may lead to increased bleeding, and concern has been raised regarding their inhibitory effect on the immune system.

So what are we to do in our daily diets? There are obvious health benefits in eating fish rich in protein, B vitamins, minerals like iron and zinc, and low saturated fat. Indeed, eating fish twice a week has been shown to reduce the risk of coronary deaths.

The fishes richest in omega-3 fatty acids include salmon, sardines, mackerel, herring, blue fish, white fish, and halibut; lesser amounts are found in rainbow trout, striped bass, shark, and swordfish. So we should learn to eat more fish in our regular daily diet, at least two times a week.

Dr. William Castelli, director of the Framingham Heart Study, is cited as saying, "If you can't be a fish, the next best thing is to eat a fish."

Overdoing Reduction in Fats: Remember the Essential Fatty Acids

It is difficult to keep up with all the changing instructions we are receiving regarding dietary fat, cholesterol, and coronary heart disease. After we got used to eating margarine and poly-unsaturated vegetable oils to replace butter and other products high in saturated fats, we were recently advised to use less margarine and to use more *monounsaturated* olive and canola oil. Generally, we were told to use all kinds of fat, only sparingly, and to eat grains and complex carbohydrates. Now we are being cautioned to be aware that too rigid a fat restriction may lead to our taking in too little of two essential fatty acids that are basic to human nutrition—*linoleic* and *linolenic* fatty acid. They cannot be manufactured by the human body but are plentiful in foods like soybeans, various nuts and seeds, and green leafy vegetables. Linoleic acid, an omega-6 fatty acid, is present in safflower oil, corn oil, cottonseed and soybean oil. Linolenic, an omega-3 fatty acid like that found in fish and fish oils, is also found in soybean and canola oil, flax seed, and purslane. Low levels of linoleic acid and linolenic acid are somehow related to coronary heart disease and there is much interest in this finding at present, but the mechanism for why this is so is not known. The interrelationship between smoking and low levels of linoleic acid, which is believed to lead to low levels of linolenic acid in the blood, is complex and yet to be worked out.

It seems reasonable at present to stay on a low-fat diet but not an entirely no-fat diet, and to eat enough green leafy vegetables, seeds, nuts, and fish until we get the next dietary guidelines from research in this field.

The experts in the field, when polled, all favor reducing the 36 percent calories from fat that most Americans consume and suggest getting below the Dietary Guidelines' 30 percent of ideal intake, even to a 25 percent level. This translates into no more than one 3-ounce serving of red meat per week, which must be about half the red meat that most Americans eat and almost a quarter of what most men eat. These experts also suggest we eat no more than three eggs a week.

Dietary Fiber

We all have become fiber conscious. In addition to all the food advice we get from publications, we are deluged by TV ads that emphasize the fiber content of a hundred cereals and breakfast foods.

We may resist this hyperbole, but the basic advice is sound. Fiber is good for us. Diets that are rich in fiber do seem to prevent and protect against constipation, diverticulosis, heart disease, and colon cancer. So far in this chapter on eating for health, I have not singled out fiber, but if you were to follow a diet that health experts stress, and which includes generous helpings of cereals, grains, vegetables, fruits, and salad, you would automatically be consuming the recommended 25 to 30 grams of fiber we ought to be eating.

What Is Dietary Fiber?

Even the experts have trouble defining terms. Dietary fiber includes all the complex plant carbohydrates that are not digested and absorbed in the small intestine. This means all the substances that enter the colon undigested. In the small intestine, almost all the food substances and most liquids and vitamins are completely absorbed. Iron is absorbed only precisely in the amount the body requires. So the undigested residues of plant foods enter the colon, whose main function in the past was considered only to absorb water and some salts.

Once fiber enters the colon, the local bacteria digest it in the process called *fermentation*, which plays a small part in the human but is terribly important in animals that subsist on plants and grains. This intestinal colonic fiber was formerly thought to be responsible for the bulk of the stool only because of the water-holding capacity of the fiber. This may not be the whole story. The bulk may be due to the increased bacterial content of the stool since the colonic organisms live off the fibrous materials (half of the normal stool is made up of bacteria).

The fiber also hastens the transit time that undigested material remains in the colon and lowers the pressure in the tail end of the colon. All these features are all to the good, and we want to aim at getting 25 to 30 grams of fiber down the intestinal tract daily. Table 3 lists the fiber content of the common foods in the American diet, their usual serving units, and the amount of fiber in grams. It is a useful guide to follow.

Now I must backtrack and add another dimension to our discussion of the colon and fiber: the nutritional role of colonic digestion of fiber and other undigested dietary components. I have said that the small bowel absorbs almost all of the nutrients that pass through it. But there is one exception. Some of the complex carbohydrates behave differently. Anywhere between 2 to 20 percent of the starch in wheat flour, rice, beans, and potatoes are not absorbed in the small bowel but pass into the colon. Even normal individuals with the necessary enzyme equipment in the small bowel may fail to process some sugars such as sucrose and lactose. So as much as 70 grams a day of unabsorbed carbohydrates enter the colon where they are absorbed directly or transformed by the colonic bacteria into the gases methane, hydrogen, and carbon dioxide. In addition, the complex carbohydrates, such as plant starches and fibers, are fermented by the intestinal bacteria into the short-chain fatty acids (SCFA): acetic, propionic, and butyric acids. These SCFA provide nutrition to the colonic lining cells, as well as increase the absorption of salt and water by the colon. The lining cells need the short-chain fatty acids for their own nutrition and to promote further absorption—additional reasons why we should maintain a high-fiber intake. So fiber plays a more complex role than was thought in the past.

Going with the Grain

In enlarging the fiber in our diet, we are urged by nutritionists to use the grain family, which for most of us is exhausted after we get past pasta and rice. But there are many other fiber-rich

Table 3. Fiber Content of Common Foods

	Serving Size	Weight (grams)	Fiber (grams)
Bread and Crackers			
Graham crackers or digestive biscuits	2 squares	14.2	1.4
Rye bread	1 slice	24	1.4
Whole-wheat or whole meal bread	1 slice	25	0.8
Whole-wheat cracker	6 crackers	19.8	2.2
Whole-wheat roll	¾ roll	21	1.2
Cereals			
All Bran, 100%	⅓ cup	28	8.4
Bran Chex	½ cup	21	4.1
Corn Bran	½ cup	21	4.4
Cornflakes	¾ cup	21	2.6
Grape Nuts flakes	⅔ cup	21	2.5
Grape Nuts	3 tbsp.	21	2.7
Oatmeal	¾ pkg.	21	2.5
Shredded wheat or Weetabix	1 piece	21	2.8
Wheat flakes	¾ cup	21	2.6
Fruit			
Apple	½ large	83	2.0
Apricot	2	72	1.4
Banana	½ medium	54	1.5
Blackberries	¾ cup	108	6.7
Cantaloupe	1 cup	160	1.6
Cherries	10 large	68	1.1
Dates, dried	2	18	1.6
Figs, dried	1 medium	20	3.7
Grapes, white	10	50	0.5
Grapefruit	½	87	0.8
Honeydew melon	1 cup	170	1.5
Orange	1 small	78	1.6
Peach	1 medium	100	2.3
Pear	½ medium	82	2.0
Pineapple	½	78	0.8
Plum	3 small	85	1.8
Prunes, dried	2	15	2.4
Raisins or Sultanas	1½ tbsp.	14	1.0

(*continued*)

Table 3. Fiber Content of Common Foods (continued)

	Serving Size	Weight (grams)	Fiber (grams)
Fruit (*continued*)			
Strawberries	1 cup	143	3.1
Tangerine	1 large	101	2.0
Watermelon	1 cup	160	1.4
Meat, Milk, Eggs			
Beef	1 oz.	28	0
Cheese	¾ oz.	21	0
Chicken/Turkey	1 oz.	28	0
Cold cuts, hot dogs	1 oz.	28	0
Eggs	3 large	99	0
Fish	2 oz.	56	0
Ice cream	1 oz.	28	0
Milk	1 cup	240	0
Pork	1 oz.	28	0
Yogurt	5 oz.	140	0
Rice			
Rice, brown (cooked)	⅓ cup	65	1.6
Rice, white (cooked)	⅓ cup	68	0.5
Leaf Vegetables			
Broccoli	½ cup	93	3.5
Brussels sprouts	½ cup	78	2.3
Cabbage	½ cup	85	2.1
Cauliflower	½ cup	90	1.6
Celery	½ cup	60	1.1
Lettuce	1 cup	55	0.8
Spinach, raw	1 cup	55	0.2
Turnip greens	½ cup	93	3.5
Root Vegetables			
Beets	½ cup	85	2.1
Carrots	½ cup	78	2.4
Potatoes, baked	½ medium	75	1.9
Radishes	½ cup	58	1.3
Sweet potatoes, baked	½ medium	75	2.1
Other Vegetables			
Beans, green	½ cup	64	2.1
Beans, string	½ cup	55	1.9

(*continued*)

Table 3. Fiber Content of Common Foods (continued)

	Serving Size	Weight (grams)	Fiber (grams)
Other Vegetables (continued)			
Cucumber	½ cup	70	1.1
Eggplant (Aubergine)	½ cup	100	2.5
Lentils, cooked	½ cup	100	3.7
Mushrooms	½ cup	35	0.9
Onions	½ cup	58	1.2
Tomatoes	1 small	100	1.5
Winter squash	½ cup	120	3.5
Zucchini squash (Courgette)	½ cup	65	2.0

Source: Based on analyses of dietary fiber by James W. Anderson, M.D., *Plant Fiber in Foods*, University of Kentucky Medical Center, 1980.

whole grains that can be added as variety to our diets, improving their taste and texture. Half a cup of cooked grains has only about 100 calories, and there is not enough fat to mention.

These other grains include couscous (grains of finely cracked wheat), bulgur (granules of dried crushed wheat), roasted buckwheat groats, and barley (usually not sold in its whole-grain version but refined as pearled barley), which, like oats, is a good source of soluble fiber and has been shown to lower blood cholesterol. Rarer grains include amaranth, quinoa, and millet. Couscous and bulgar can be found in many supermarkets, but the others—amaranth, quinoa, and millet—can only be found in health food stores. All of these grains go well with soups and salads.

Vegetables and Fruits

Vegetables and fruits are the current good guys in nutrition, and all published authorities favor eating at least five servings of fruits or vegetables daily. Privately, the experts feel that seven a day would be better. Diets rich in these two groups reduce the risk of certain cancers, including cancer of the lung, colon, breast, cervix, esophagus, oral cavity, stomach, bladder, pancreas, and ovaries. The group singled out as most beneficial are the cruciferous vegetables—broccoli, cabbage, cauliflower, brussels sprouts, and kale. Researchers believe the powerful effect of these vegetables may be related in part to their content of antioxidants and vitamins—especially beta-carotene and vitamins C and E. Sweet potatoes, spinach, cantaloupe, string beans, citrus fruits, and the lowly potato are also good sources of the antioxidants.

Can Food Protect Us Against Disease?

There is a growing body of evidence that eating a diet rich in vegetables and fruits may help prevent digestive diseases, cancer, and heart disease. Some recent research has focused on a compound of broccoli called sulforaphane that blocks the growth of blood tissue tumors in animals treated with a cancer-causing toxin.

Sulforaphane is a member of a class of chemicals called *isothiocyanates* that increases the body's output of enzymes and that are able to detoxify carcinogens. The isothiocyanates have no nutritional value like vitamins, fiber, minerals, and vegetables, but they may be the protective element of a plant-based diet. An intensive search is now under way in an effort to identify more of this class of substances in vegetable plants. Among those suspected of protecting us from diseases are limonene in citrus fruits, allium compounds in garlic and onions, isoflavones in beans, and eleagic acid in grapes.

The Antioxidants

Recent nutritional research has focused on certain substances, including vitamins C and E and beta-carotene, which are collectively known as the *antioxidants*. These vitamins fight free oxygen radicals in the tissues that are harmful to blood vessels and muscles. Some studies indicate that people who eat foods high in antioxidants have lower rates of cancer and heart disease. The U.S. Recommended Daily Allowance (RDA) for these substances as proposed by the Food and Drug Administration are 60 milligrams for vitamin C, 30 International Units (or IUs) of vitamin E, and no recommended daily dosage is advised for beta-carotene. But the feeling is growing that one ought to take more than these levels. Some authorities have favored supplements, whereas others have stressed that the increased amounts be obtained from foods, especially fruits and vegetables. Although some recent studies have quelled the enthusiasm for these supplements, most researchers favor a daily intake of food rich in the antioxidants.

The Role of Antioxidants in the Diet

Almost everyone you know who is "health conscious" is taking supplements of vitamins C and E and beta-carotene to guard against insult to their body from within and without. They want to guard against such influences as cigarette smoke and air pollution, as well as fatty diets and cancer. By taking these supplements, labeled the antioxidants, individuals hope they are safeguarding their health.

How do these substances work? It is believed that they are capable of blocking the harmful effects of the highly reactive oxidizing substances—the free radicals—that arise from our normal metabolism and the onslaughts of the external environment. These free oxygen radicals can damage blood vessels and possibly can stimulate cancer-causing substances in the colon and breast. The ongoing studies suggest a beneficial role for the antioxidants, but the story is far from complete.

Vitamin E I single out vitamin E here because it is difficult to get sufficient amounts of this vitamin in a low-fat diet or one suitable for individuals with heart disease. Thus most experts suggest a daily supplement of vitamin E. But what are the benefits of taking large doses of vitamin E?

Vitamin E, known as alpha tocopherol, helps form red blood cells, muscles, and other tissues, and prevents the oxidation and destruction of vitamin A and essential fatty acids when taken in usual low doses. When taken in higher doses, up to 100 IUs, it acts as a drug, and no longer a nutrient.

At levels not obtained by diet alone, at forty times the calculated nutritional needed amount (which is 30 IUs), it may help prevent coronary heart disease and has been reported to reduce the risk of heart attacks by 75 percent. It prevents the oxidation of LDL cholesterol (the low-density lipoprotein, the so-called bad cholesterol), which clogs our arteries. It may also help persons with hardening of the arteries in the legs, may prevent clotting, and, when combined with aspirin, is more effective than aspirin alone in combatting heart disease. Against cancer, the evidence is less convincing, but work in animals has been promising.

The verdict is not clear, however, for many human disorders. Vitamin E may interfere with clotting, and thus may cause bleeding, and in some individuals it may raise blood pressure. These are reasons for caution in the use of any megadoses.

On the other hand, some individuals may need increased amounts of vitamin E. These individuals include those engaging in heavy exercise, cigarette smokers, and those exposed to excessive air pollutants. Other evidence reveals that consuming a high-fat diet or taking fish oil supplements may use up the body's stores of vitamin E. Moreover, most vegetable oils and margarines supply the wrong type of tocopherols and ironically increase the body's need for vitamin E. Olive oil, however, is rich in the tocopherols that are beneficial. But, again, individuals on very low-fat diets may not consume enough vitamin E in their foods and may need to take a supplement.

What Is Folic Acid?

It has been known for many years that folic acid—a B vitamin, also called *folate*—is essential in the formation of hemoglobin, part of the red blood cells. Lack of folic acid leads to a particular form of anemia, the megaloblastic form, which creates large partially empty red blood cells. Since folate can cure pernicious anemia, but fails to treat the neurological difficulties of vitamin B12 deficiency associated with pernicious anemia, there has been considerable anxiety about fortifying foods with folic acid, and indeed the recommended daily dose of 40 milligrams was lowered in 1989 to half (20 milligrams a day).

But more recent research shows that the adult daily recommended dose should be at least 400 micrograms. In our ordinary diets, folic acid is mainly derived from green leafy vegetables, but other foods contain folic acid as well. Natural foods, however, may be a somewhat less reliable source of folic acid than supplements or foods fortified with folate because folic acid can be destroyed by processing and cooking. And its absorption can be interfered with by alcohol and intestinal ailments. Recent studies of the American diet reveal that our intake of this important vitamin is quite low in the general population, which derives most of its folic acid from liver, fruits, fortified cereals, nuts and seeds, and beans. For most Americans, the chief source of folate is orange juice, a cup of which may contain anywhere between 75 to 100 micrograms. The next leading source is white bread, which contains 8 to 10 micrograms per slice. Whole wheat bread supplies three times that amount.

But the current emphasis on folic acid concerns its possible value in preventing heart disease and some cancers, and several researchers are now focusing their attention on the relationship between low-folate levels and other disease. The way in which low-folate levels can lead to heart disease is complex and needs much more work, but it seems the current levels of folate considered normal may be too low to prevent heart attacks. A sim-

Table 4A. Dietary Sources of Folate

Barley	Orange juice
Beans	Peas
Brewer's yeast	Rice
Endive	Soybeans
Fruits	Split peas
Garbanzo beans (chick-peas)	Sprouts
Green leafy vegetables	Uncooked vegetable greens
Lentils	Wheat
Liver	Wheat germ
Most animal products	Whole wheat
Oranges	

ilar picture seems to be emerging with regard to low blood folate levels and the presence of benign tumors in the colon, called *adenomas*, which are the precursors of cancer in that organ. In animals prone to develop cancers of the colon, added doses of folic acid seemed to slow the development of cancer. Low blood levels of folic acid have also been linked to cervical cancer due to a cancer-causing strain of human papilloma virus. And the list is growing longer: low levels of folic acid may increase the risk of cancer of the lung, esophagus, and breast.

These cancer-prevention studies will need to be greatly expanded, but it is clear from what we know now that 400 micrograms of folate is a good daily target. Certainly, pregnant women need twice that amount to prevent neurological abnormalities in their offspring, and nursing women need even more folate.

The accompanying Tables 4A, B list the dietary sources of folic acid and vitamin B12. To be used in our bodies, folic acid in food must be stripped of glutamic acid and converted to folate in its active form. Thus the supplements and fortified foods that contain the more active form may be more easily absorbed than the natural form of folate.

Recent research reveals yet another reason for paying attention to the folic acid in our diets. It has been known for a long time that children with a rare genetic disease called *homocys-*

Table 4B. Dietary Sources of Vitamin B12[a]

Meat
Organ meats
Cheese, yogurt, etc.
Eggs
Milk
Milk products
Fish
Shellfish

[a]"Anything that walks, swims, or flies contains B12. Nothing that grows out of the ground contains B12." (Victor Herbert, M.D.)

teinuria, who have very high blood levels of an amino acid called *homocysteine*, often showed evidence of clogged arteries (atherosclerosis), which leads to stroke or heart disease.

Long neglected by investigators, this disease may shed light on adults who have high blood levels of homocysteine. These individuals may be at risk of developing atherosclerosis, stroke, and heart disease. For some, this may be based on a genetic predisposition, as it is with children with this condition.

But where does folic acid come in? It seems folic acid can reduce such damage, at least in experimental animals, by reducing the blood level of homocysteine to a safe range. In fact, we can reduce high levels of this amino acid in the blood more easily with folate than with fiber diets and medicine. To increase folic acid in our diet, turn to fresh fruits and vegetables, especially the dark green leafy ones, orange juice, or take folic acid supplements.

The Key Minerals

Iron

Iron is the important part of hemoglobin, which transports oxygen from the lungs to organs and muscles in the body. We depend entirely on our diet for iron, and menstruating women especially need a rich source of iron in their foods. But many of us can obtain the needed dietary requirements of iron from our diet alone. Vegetables, beans and peas, grain products, and small amounts of fish, poultry, or meat (Table 5) can supply most people with the necessary daily supply of iron. Adding vitamin C to the diet will increase the absorption of iron contained in beans, grains, and green leafy vegetables while in the bowel. Vitamin C can be obtained from many foods, especially potatoes, with their skins left on, or tomatoes, as well as citrus fruits and citrus juices.

While we are discussing iron in the diet, it might be a good idea to present some recent concerns about iron and heart disease. Although an early report from Finland showed that high levels of blood iron double the risk of heart disease in men, recent studies have failed to confirm this finding; we need not concern ourselves with this factor. As I have already pointed out, the body absorbs iron in the upper gut only as needed, and menstruating women, of course, lose blood and therefore iron monthly.

Calcium

A second important mineral is *calcium*, which plays a part in bone metabolism and growth and is clinically related to osteoporosis, the weakness of bones which is prevalent in postmenopausal women. The U.S. daily minimal requirement for calcium has been 1000 milligrams, or one gram daily, but now the National Institutes of Health recommends 1500 milligrams of calcium daily for postmenopausal women. This suggested amount requires that these women take a daily supplement of calcium in addition to the calcium derived from their diet. Growing boys and girls may need to do the same. Recently, new studies of calcium requirements insist that the former daily recommendations be increased. Children and young adults, eleven to twenty-four years old, should take between 1200 to 1500 mil-

Table 5. Iron Content of Foods

	Serving Size	Iron (in milligrams)
Meat, Fish, Poultry		
Beef, roast	3.0 oz.	6.1
Beef liver (fried)	3.5 oz.	5.7
Beef sirloin (lean, cooked)	3.5 oz.	3.4
Blood sausage	2.0 oz.	1.0
Calves' liver	3.5 oz.	14.2
Chicken, dark meat	3.5 oz.	1.3
Chicken, light meat	3.5 oz.	1.1
Chicken liver (simmered)	3.5 oz.	8.5
Clam (raw meat)	3.5 oz.	3.0
Flounder or sole (baked)	3.5 oz.	0.4
Ham (canned)	3.5 oz.	0.8
Hamburger (lean, cooked)	3.5 oz.	2.1
Lamb, leg (roasted)	3.5 oz.	2.2
Lamb chop (lean, without bone)	3.5 oz.	1.8
Liverwurst, pork	1.0 oz.	1.8
Oysters, eastern (raw meat)	3.5 oz.	6.5
Pork chop	3.5 oz.	4.5
Pork liver (braised)	3.5 oz.	17.9
Pork loin (broiled, lean)	3.5 oz.	0.9
Salmon (red, baked)	3.0 oz.	0.6
Sardines	3.5 oz.	3.0
Shrimp (cooked)	3.0 oz.	2.5
Shrimp (raw)	3.5 oz.	1.8
Tuna (light, oil-packed)	3.5 oz.	1.9
Tuna (white, water-packed)	3.5 oz.	0.7
Turkey, dark meat	3.5 oz.	2.3
Turkey, light meat	3.5 oz.	1.4
Veal cutlet	3.5 oz.	3.0
Beans		
Black beans	½ cup	1.4
Chick-peas	½ cup	2.4
Kidney beans	½ cup	2.8
Lentils	½ cup	2.1
Lima beans	½ cup	3.0
Pinto beans	½ cup	2.7

(*continued*)

Table 5. Iron Content of Foods (continued)

	Serving Size	Iron (in milligrams)
Grain Products		
Bagel	1	1.8
Bulgur, uncooked	¼ cup	2.4
Cheerios	1 oz.	4.5
Cornflakes	1 oz.	1.8
Farina	¾ cup	0.9
Grits	¾ cup	1.2
Oatmeal (fortified)	¾ cup	6.3
Oatmeal (nonfortified)	¾ cup	1.2
Pasta, enriched	2.0 oz.	2.2
Rice, cooked (enriched)	½ cup	0.9
Rice, cooked (brown)	½ cup	0.4
Rye bread	1 slice	0.7
Saltine cracker	4	0.5
Total cereal	1 cup	21.0
Wheat germ (plain, toasted)	1 tbsp.	0.6
White enriched bread	1 slice	0.8
Whole-wheat bread	1 slice	0.8
Nuts and Seeds		
Almonds (whole)	1 oz.	1.0
Cashews, oil-roasted	1 oz.	1.2
Cashews, dry-roasted	1 oz.	1.7
Peanut butter	1 tbsp.	0.3
Peanuts, oil-roasted	1 oz.	0.5
Peanuts, dry-roasted	1 oz.	0.9
Pistachios	1 oz.	1.9
Pumpkin seeds	1 oz.	4.2
Sesame seeds, hulled	1 oz.	0.6
Sunflower seeds	1 oz.	0.7
Walnuts	1 oz.	0.7
Vegetables		
Acorn squash (baked)	½ cup	1.0
Asparagus (fresh, cooked)	½ cup	0.6
Bean sprouts (mung), raw	½ cup	0.5
Beets (boiled)	½ cup	0.5
Beet greens (boiled)	½ cup	1.4
Broccoli (cooked, chopped)	½ cup	0.9

(*continued*)

Table 5. Iron Content of Foods (continued)

	Serving Size	Iron (in milligrams)
Vegetables (continued)		
Brussels sprouts (cooked)	½ cup	0.9
Collard greens	1 cup	1.7
Corn (boiled)	½ cup	0.5
Corn grits	¼ cup	1.4
Green peas, frozen	½ cup	1.3
Hash-brown potatoes	½ cup	1.2
Kale (cooked)	½ cup	0.6
Mushrooms, cooked	½ cup	1.4
Mustard greens	½ cup	2.5
Parsley (raw, chopped)	½ cup	1.9
Potato (baked with skin)	1 large	2.8
Pumpkin, canned	½ cup	0.7
Snow peas, boiled	½ cup	1.6
Spinach	1 cup	0.8
Sweet pepper, raw	½ cup	0.6
Tomato, raw	1 medium	0.6
Tomato juice	½ cup	0.7
Tomato sauce	½ cup	1.0
Turnip greens (fresh, cooked)	½ cup	0.6
Turnip greens (frozen, cooked)	½ cup	1.6
Fruit		
Apricots (dried)	8 halves	2.5
Avocado, California	½ fruit	1.0
Blackberries, raw	1 cup	0.8
Blackstrap molasses	1 tbsp.	5.0
Cantaloupe	½ melon	0.6
Light molasses	1 tbsp.	1.2
Orange	1 medium	1.0
Prune juice	½ cup	1.5
Prunes	5 fruits	1.0
Raisins	¼ cup	0.8
Raspberries, raw	1 cup	0.7

Source: U.S. Department of Agriculture; adapted from V. Herbert, C. J. Subak-Sharp, eds., *The Mount Sinai School of Medicine's Complete Book of Nutrition*, New York, St. Martin's Press, 1990.

Table 6. Calcium-Rich Foods

Item	Serving Size	Calcium (in milligrams)
Sardines, with bones	3 oz.	372
Skim milk	1 cup	296
Whole milk	1 cup	288
Yogurt	1 cup	272
Swiss cheese	1 oz.	262
Cheddar cheese	1 oz.	213
American cheese	1 oz.	198
Oysters	¼ cup	170
Salmon, canned with bones	3 oz.	167
Collard greens	½ cup	145
Cottage cheese, creamed	½ cup	116
Spinach, cooked	½ cup	106
Ice cream	½ cup	97
Mustard greens, cooked	½ cup	97
Corn muffin	2 medium	90
Cottage cheese, dry curd	½ cup	90
Kale, cooked	½ cup	74
Broccoli, cooked	½ cup	68
Orange	1 medium	54

Source: Based on data in *Agriculture Handbooks,* Nos. 8 and 456. Other foods high in calcium include almonds, bok choy (spoon cabbage), dandelion greens, dried fruits (most), legumes, molasses (black strap), okra, rutabaga, and turnip greens.

ligrams; and men twenty-five years and older, as well as women ages twenty-five to fifty, should take 1000 milligrams.

Since most of us rely on dairy products as our main sources of calcium, it is important to select low-fat varieties to be sure your fat intake isn't increased in your effort to maintain recommended calcium levels. (For dietary calcium sources, see Table 6.)

Aside from dairy products and broccoli, the majority of American diets do not contain other food sources rich in calcium—kale, collard greens, sardines, and okra are not common staples in the American diet but do have plenty of calcium. Many of my patients avoid dairy products because of the high-fat content; yet low-fat dairy products are readily available and may supply adequate amounts of calcium. Skimmed and low-fat milk, nonfat buttermilk, nonfat plain yogurt or with fruit, reduced-fat sour cream, and reduced-fat ricotta are other good calcium sources. Some recipes that take advantage of these ingredients might approve of a risotto made with Swiss chard and Parmigiano-Reggiano cheese, tofu and broccoli, or potato salads made with buttermilk rather than the usual high-fat mayonnaise.

Zinc

Zinc, which is usually included in many multivitamin supplements, especially in preparations for the elderly, may not be entirely innocent according to a recent study from Boston, which suggested that it might hasten or add to the deterioration of patients with Alzheimer's disease. Some practitioners recommend zinc in megadoses for macular degeneration of the retina, but given the recent finding that links zinc to Alzheimer's, caution has now been suggested.

So What Supplements Do I Really Need?

All authors agree that it would be far better to get our vitamins and other nutritients from our diet rather than supplements, but most experts admit that many individuals prefer to get some assurances from their multivitamins.

As I have already mentioned, beta-carotene, vitamin C, and vitamin E are recommended by most experts. The natural form of vitamin E seems to be better absorbed by the body, so you might look at the label on your vitamin bottle—alpha tocopherol is the natural form.

Supplements high in beta-carotene are better than those high in vitamin A, since beta-carotene is converted to vitamin A in the body and is the desired antioxidant. Large doses of vitamin A can be toxic, and the maximum dose considered safe is 500 IUs per day. There are a few other cases where supplements of vitamins may be necessary, especially calcium.

Most of us get our vitamin D from exposure to the sun, except during the period from October to March, and postmenopausal women should consume 400 IUs daily of vitamin D to avoid bone loss.

Vegetarians who consume no animal or dairy products must take supplements of vitamin B12 daily.

And trace elements, *selenium* and *chromium*, are often omitted from multivitamin pills, but should be part of a daily supplement. At least 50 but no more than 200 milligrams each of selenium and chromium is recommended. Both elements are needed, but we just don't know enough to specify an exact amount.

Three Food Elements That May Cause Problems

Salt (Sodium)

The popularly held feeling is that salt is bad for our health. This is clearly the case for half of the sixty million people in the United States with high blood pressure. The National Research Council advises all Americans to reduce their daily salt intake to less than 6 grams a day (about one-and-a-half teaspoonfuls)— 2400 milligrams of sodium. This is about half the current intake of most people. And while 6 grams seems very little, many nutritional experts would suggest a reduction of salt intake to 4.5 grams of salt daily. The real benefits of sodium reduction accrue to people with high blood pressure or those at risk of its development, as well as the overweight and the elderly. African Americans have a higher than average genetic risk of salt-sensitive high blood pressure and must be particularly careful about sodium intake.

Sugar

Sugar, too, has a bad reputation, mainly because it provides "empty calories" that contain energy but little of nutritional value. Americans eat large amounts of calories derived from candy, sweetened snacks and drinks, and this clearly contributes to our weight gain. At present, Americans get 11 percent of their daily caloric intake from sugars and are advised to reduce this amount to around 5 percent of calories. Yet many of us who have a sweet tooth know this is difficult. The real risk of sugar is its contribution to obesity and overweightness, and probably, equally important, its contribution to tooth decay.

Coffee

Another topic often in the news is coffee, a beverage used throughout the world. While the pros and cons are still being debated, we know several things about this popular stimulant. Boiled coffee contributes to elevated blood cholesterol levels, while filtered coffee does not. Unfortunately, the original studies on coffee were done on the percolated form, which is rarely used today. Recently, instant coffee has been exonerated from harmful effects.

I discuss the role of coffee-containing foods and beverages in Chapter 4, but here let me add that coffee may contribute to an irregular heartbeat in some individuals.

Alcohol

I discuss the issue of alcohol in the diet of specific gastrointestinal disorders as I proceed through the gastrointestinal tract in Part II of this book.

Here I want to touch on the question of alcohol intake in general. Products of the vine have been enjoyed by men and women ever since we were expelled from the Garden of Eden, but its role in our health presents us with a dilemma.

At least thirty-five careful studies confirm the fact that moderate alcohol consumption (equal to two drinks a day for men and one drink for women) is associated with a lower risk of coronary heart disease. However, at more than that level the rate of disease and death increases markedly.

The beneficial effects of moderate drinking are ascribed to alcohol's ability to increase the high-density lipoproteins (the "good" cholesterol, called HDL) in the blood, which removes cholesterol from the arteries. Alcohol also decreases the tendency of the blood to clot and may act as an antioxidant.

More than three drinks a day for men and women, however, may increase cancer, cirrhosis, high blood pressure, and stroke, as well as different kinds of heart disease, disturbances in the heart rhythm, along with heart muscle degeneration (cardiomyopathy). For women, the added risk also includes increased risk of cancer of the breast, as well as damage to the fetus if they are pregnant, and both sexes run the risk of alcoholism, especially if they have a family history of this disorder.

Because of the difference between men and women in the way alcohol is metabolized, moderate drinking in women means only one drink of alcohol daily.

So you see there are real risks in advising patients to start drinking alcohol to avoid coronary heart disease. In general, there seems to be no difference between hard liquors, beer, and wine. It's the alcohol content that matters, although red wine has been advocated in the Mediterranean diet. One drink equals 12 ounces of beer, 5 ounces of wine, or 1.5 ounces of spirits.

I do not advise nondrinkers to start drinking alcohol to avoid heart disease and certainly not those with a family history of alcoholism. Women must understand the increased risk of breast cancer, and their family history of this disease is important to take into consideration. Thus, women have little to gain from alcohol and much to lose. Drinking during pregnancy is entirely prohibited by all experts.

For men who are moderate drinkers and who have had a heart attack, I see little value in continuing to drink.

Given all that we know at this point, it is interesting to see what the new Dietary Guidelines for 1996 suggest regarding alcohol consumption. Published every five years by the U.S. Department of Agriculture and the Department of Health and Human Services, the guidelines argue that alcohol has some healthful advantages. But they suggest no increase in the amount of alcohol that may be taken: one drink a day for women, and two drinks at most for men.

Garlic

Garlic has enjoyed a long history in the cuisines of the world and has been touted in folklore for centuries as being good for our health. Recent studies seem to bear this out. The valuable part of garlic does not depend on the substance that gives the odor to garlic, the allium. Other members of the allium family also contain the active ingredient that seems beneficial. Onions, shallots, leeks, scallions, and chives are all part of the allium family. And all these products, whether cooked, dried, powdered, or extracted with oil or water, are beneficial. Researchers have found that garlic and its relatives are rich sources of sulphur-containing compounds that are able to lower blood pressure. Garlic may also lower the triglycerides in the blood and reduce the stickiness of platelets, perhaps even more than aspirin. In an Iowa study, garlic intake lowered the incidence of colon cancer, and in a study done in China, garlic was linked to a lower incidence of stomach cancer. So it would seem prudent to include some garlic, whether in powder or other forms, in our diet without going overboard.

This chapter has focused on eating for health without concern for the individual with disorders of the gastrointestinal tract and its associated glands, the liver and pancreas. Now it is time to turn to those who have specific digestive problems.

II

GOOD
FOOD
FOR
BAD
STOMACHS

* * *

When we turn to discuss the role of food in disorders of the digestive tract, we need to be clear about what we really know. We all are interested in the role diet may play in causing a disorder. But clear-cut and established cases are few, but striking, in their importance. If a newborn baby lacks the proper enzyme systems, then it will develop the disease called phenylketonuria if the diet contains any phenylketones. If an individual's intestines are defective and contain no *lactase*—the enzyme that digests lactose, the sugar of milk—the person will be unable to digest milk or milk products. If an individual is born with or develops the disorder known as gluten enteropathy, then he or she will be unable to digest any gluten in the diet (from wheat, rye, oats, or perhaps barley). If the ileum is diseased, disordered, or removed surgically, then that would lead to trouble in absorbing vitamin B12, some forms of fat, and lead to an increase in oxalate in the urine, which leads to kidney stones. These illustrative cases seem fairly straightforward.

Another group of problems arises if the diet is deficient in certain substances. Vitamin C cannot be synthesized by the human organism, and if the diet is deficient in C, the patient develops scurvy, even in the twentieth century or the twenty-first.

But consider this situation: Cancer of the colon is seen less frequently in individuals whose diets are rich in fruits and vegetables, but we do not know what this diet contains that protects the patient. Recent studies have singled out the vitamin content (beta-carotene, the precursor of vitamin A) and antioxidants such as vitamins C or E. But the possibility may exist that these people eating less vegetables and fruit are eating more of other substances which might be harmful to the colon. We just don't have all the facts yet.

And there are the problems that arise in the area of treating intestinal conditions. What do we need to add to the diet to treat constipation and diverticulosis—usually bran and fiber. What substances in the diet should we do without? All fruits and vegetables in the case of diarrheal disorders. What substance do we add to the diet in the presence of anemia? What diet do we use in gluten malabsorption, or for hyperoxaluria and kidney stones due to increased oxalate in the urine?

This part of the book will describe what we do know about the role of food in the health of the GI tract. We start with ulcers, move to the gallbladder and pancreas, describe the dietary approach to malabsorption, food allergies and intolerances. We cannot avoid discussing the ubiquitous irritable bowel syndrome, constipation, and diarrhea. Then we enter the colon with its diverticula and diverticulitis, the inflammatory bowel diseases (Crohn's and ulcerative colitis), as well as cancer of the colon and its forerunners.

4

✻ ✻ ✻

THE ULCER
ENSEMBLE

L et's start with the upper intestinal tract and consider its in-flammatory and ulcerative disorders: heartburn and peptic esophagitis, gastric and duodenal ulcer, and gastritis. I begin here not only because the problems originate in the first portion of the gastrointestinal tract, but because they probably represent the largest group of disorders from which we suffer.

Heartburn and Peptic Esophagitis—Acid in the Gullet

Heartburn is that annoying, uncomfortable, burning discomfort just behind the breastbone, which may also reach up as high as the back of the throat. Closely aligned to it is the discomfort and the pain of *esophagitis*, also felt along the same route. In both complaints, individuals experience reflux of stomach contents and acid into the lower portion of the esophagus, which have gotten past the esophageal sphincter muscles of the lower swallowing tube—the guardians and gatekeepers that prevent the lower section of the esophagus from being invaded by these irritants. We will experience heartburn when acid gets into the esophagus and will develop esophagitis if this reflux occurs often enough to result in inflammation, and even at times ulceration, of the esophageal lining walls.

Why the sphincters let down their guard still remains an incompletely resolved problem. We used to put all the blame on a hiatal hernia in this area, but the mere presence of a hernia does not explain the periodic relaxation of the lower esophageal sphincter muscles. It is the presence of the acid that causes the mischief, but one does not need a large amount of acid, just a small amount will do. Indeed, those of us who have heartburn or esophagitis are not necessarily making larger quantities of acid than others free of the disorder and we are not oversecretors.

With reflux, our dietary habits and customary food intake can make a difference. Obviously, making less acid would help, but of equal importance, the acid must exit from the stomach promptly by the regular emptying machinery. We must arrange somehow to have as little acid as possible remaining in the stomach to be refluxed into the esophagus to solve this problem.

Let us consider first *how* we eat or should eat with this condition before we discuss *what* we should eat. In addition to the chemistry of our food, the *size* of the meal plays a crucial part in these conditions. The cells of the stomach lining are stimulated to pour forth the acid they manufacture—hydrochloric acid—when the stomach is distended and the walls stretched. So the larger the bulk of food eaten, the more likely the stomach is to be stretched taut. Given this machinery, we need to balance the volume of food eaten more evenly between our three customary meals. It makes little sense to have a scanty breakfast, gulp down a hasty sandwich at lunch, and fill the stomach at dinner with a terribly large amount of food.

When we are in the upright position during the day, the stomach regularly empties its contents into the upper intestine through its lower end, the pyloric canal. The typical meal of mixed food contents requires about three hours to be moved completely out of the stomach, taking ninety minutes for the first half—from the stomach into the small intestine. Ordinarily, as we eat sitting up, very little gets back into the esophagus by reflux. The liquid contents of the stomach cannot flow uphill. However, if we lie down, the food in the stomach of a partially digested meal may move backward into the esophagus. The best advice I can give is not to lie down or go to sleep with a full stomach shortly after eating a meal. Furthermore, if we fill the stomach with carbonated beverages, they release their dissolved carbon dioxide and further distend the stomach. Seeking an exit from the stomach and rising to the higher part of the stomach, the cardia, these beverages release this gas into the esophagus. A belch is simply the reflux of gas or air from the stomach into the swallowing tube.

So far, so good. But what should we put into the stomach if heartburn and esophagitis is the main problem, especially when there is no associated stomach inflammation or ulcer formation to complicate the picture. Obviously, we should not add any acid to our stomach contents. Indeed, most people with this complaint have already discovered that acid citrus fruits should be avoided since they contain ascorbic acid (vitamin C) as well as acetic acid. This list also includes vinegar or salad dressings containing vinegar. In this case, we must take care not to develop the deficiency of vitamin C known as scurvy, but we can get enough vitamin C from fruits and vegetables in our regular diet and a small pill supplement.

Caffeine

Caffeine intake is important for both heartburn sufferers and those with esophagitis, since caffeine is a very strong stimulant of acid (we once used caffeine as a method of stimulating the stomach to test stomach acidity). Caffeine-containing drinks must be avoided: coffee, tea, cocoa, hot chocolate—as well as over-the-counter headache pills and pills to keep us awake which also contain caffeine. We live in a world filled with caffeine (Table 7), so it won't be easy to avoid it entirely. But you must try.

Alcohol

Men and women have enjoyed fermented brews for eons, but we have learned that these beverages stimulate the gastric juices while they lubricate the flow of conversation. Yet, despite these favorable features, alcohol should be avoided with these reflux conditions. Not because it stimulates acid (in fact, alcohol is a rather poor stimulant of gastric juice), but because it irritates tissue that is already inflamed. Why would we pour alcohol over the inflamed tissues of the esophagus? We wouldn't pour alcohol over a tissue wound anywhere else in the body. For the moderate drinker who enjoys one to two drinks a day, this is not a life sentence. When the esophagus heals and stays healed for a significant amount of time (three to six months), then the restriction can be lifted. However, drinking more than two drinks a day for men and more than one for women is inadvisable for those recovering from reflux conditions, or indeed in any healthy diet.

Protein: The Building Blocks of Tissues

In the stomach, protein—animal products including meat, dairy products, egg whites, and fish and the protein content of vegetables, grains, and fruits—is a double agent. The products of protein digestion that begins in the stomach and the amino acids that result stimulate the secretion of acid. They are probably the most important chemical stimulants of acid secretion in the stomach. Yet protein also acts as a buffer as well, since it is *amphoteric*—that is, proteins stimulate acids and yet neutralize acids at the same time. So their good and bad qualities balance each other out. There is no need to worry about our protein intake. Americans eat somewhat more than the U.S. Recommended Daily Allowance of 65 grams. Nutritional experts tell us not to fuss over our protein intake in general, and I agree in the present context.

Fats and Oils

Fats and oils slow down and inhibit the secretion of acids, so why don't we concentrate on them for the treatment of upper esophagitis and heartburn? Mainly because Americans eat too much fat already and derive too large a fraction of their daily calories from fat. Many of us are already in danger of raising our LDLs, or low-density lipoproteins, which are what clogs our arteries. These products are forbidden in the diet of individuals with coronary artery disease. In addition, fats slow down gastric emptying, and we certainly want to get as much of the acid out of the stomach and into the small intestine as quickly as possible, rather than increasing the time in which the gastric contents remain in the esophagus.

Fiber

There is no reason to reduce the intake of fiber in instances of heartburn and esophagitis, except perhaps in just one instance. That is the situation in which repeated episodes of untreated esophagitis have left a scarred, narrowed gullet and a strictured area, one with a narrowed lumen. In this case, the roughage of your diet may get stuck in the gullet.

Effects of Specific Foods and Drinks on the Lower Esophageal Sphincter

A variety of foods increases the likelihood of reflux of contents from the stomach into the esophagus. They include alcohol, fats, large bulky meals, coffee (whether caffeinated or decaffeinated), tea, cola drinks, all of which lower esophageal sphincter pressure. Chocolate, especially chocolate syrup, produces an immediate drop in pressure in the sphincter muscles, which may last for up to an hour. Peppermint and spearmint also lower sphincter pressure.

Interestingly enough, whole milk produces a slight drop in pressure that is in contrast to nonfat milk which produces a real rise in pressure that may last for an hour. Orange juice and tomato juice do little to sphincter pressure. Drugs can also reduce lower esophageal sphincter pressure. The list includes anticholinergic drugs (like atropine or belladonna), theophylline, and relaxants like Diazapin® or calcium channel blockers such as nefetamine (Procardia®). If at all possible, these should be avoided.

What about Food Sensitivities?

We all learn that certain foods will give us heartburn, so we must consider that the direct effect of these on the esophagus has little to do with the sphincters and sphincter pressure. Coffee, orange juice, and spicy tomato drinks appear on many individuals' lists, and they all have been blamed for their acidity.

One must remember that sensitivity of the esophagus to these substances varies from person to person. One group of individuals are highly sensitive to acid solutions being dripped into their esophaguses (the so-called Bernstein test), while others seem to tolerate this maneuver with no distress. Coffee, oranges, and a Bloody Mary mix without the alcohol cause heartburn in acid-sensitive individuals but not in others. Yet it is not entirely due to acidity because they still cause heartburn even when the acid of these substances is neutralized. Thus acidity alone cannot explain why different individuals regularly get heartburn after different acidic meals only after certain specific substances are eaten or drunk.

Some investigators have suggested that it is the concentration of substances in a particular drink that causes the heartburn, not the acidity. Apple juice, grape juice, as well as orange juice, are highly concentrated solutions as is the liquid portion of pizza preparations.

A Dietary Approach to Heartburn and Peptic Esophagitis

Your basic diet should be founded on the kinds of foods I have outlined in Chapter 3. With these conditions, a reduction of fat intake is especially important because it lowers the pressure of the esophageal sphincter and delays gastric emptying. If we drink milk, it should be a low-fat preparation. We ought to avoid coffee and caffeine-containing drinks, especially dark chocolate that also lowers sphincter pressure and favors reflux. Orange juice, grapefruit juice, and grape juice should be avoided until healing takes place and symptoms clear. Alcohol is an absolute no-no. "Spicy" drinks and foods can cause heartburn in susceptible individuals.

But the way we eat this healthy diet is also important. Our food should be evenly divided between our three meals over the course of the day, avoiding overfilling the stomach at the end of a tiring day. The stomach needs time to empty its contents, so try to give yourself at least three to three and one-half hours after a meal before retiring at bedtime. One should also try to sleep with the chest higher than the abdomen because acids cannot travel uphill.

The Role of Medication

Will Diet Alone Do the Trick?

For some individuals, yes. For many, no. Long-standing heart-burn and the inflammatory changes of peptic esophagitis may require more potent medicines to stop acid secretion (a hista-mine II blocker, such as Tagamet, Zantac, Axaid, and Pepcid), which are now over-the-counter products. The newest that are more potent include omeprazole (Prilosec® in the U.S., Losec elsewhere in the world), and lansoprazole (Prevacid®). For a few individuals antacids alone (Mylanta, Maalox, Riopan, etc.) may be enough. Others may require drugs to tighten the sphinc-ter and hasten gastric emptying (Propulsid®).

How Long Must We Follow This Program?

The obvious answer is until all the symptoms clear and the tis-sues of the inflamed esophagus heal. It may take only a short period of time or several weeks for the symptoms of heartburn and pain to clear, but the inflammatory process will require much more time. I urge you to follow the strict program for at least three months; it would be unwise to stop earlier just be-cause you feel better. This is a common excuse and the com-monest reason why symptoms recur.

Peptic Ulcer Disease

It is convenient to discuss the role of diet in duodenal and gas-tric ulcers together under the heading of peptic ulcer. This as-sumes that these two varieties of ulcer are similar and are caused by a similar localized self-digestion of an area of the stomach or duodenum by the acid-peptic fluid secreted by the stomach lining. Indeed, the slogan, "No acid—no ulcer," has been repeated for almost the entire twentieth century.

However, workers in this field have always been aware that there are differences between the ulcer in the stomach (gastric ulcers) and the ulcer in the duodenum. Patients with duodenal ulcers secrete more acid and their ulcers occur at an earlier age than those with gastric ulcers. The aspirin-like drugs (nonsteroidal anti-inflammatory drugs, NSAIDs) play a greater role in stomach ulcers than duodenal ulcers. Finally, all clinicians know that one must be sure that the ulcer of the stomach is benign and not the first indication of cancer.

Now we are in the midst of a real revolution of our thinking about peptic ulcer. We have been turned around a complete 180 degrees by the pioneer work of an Australian investigator, Bernard Marshall, and his coworker J. R. Warner. Just ten years ago they announced their concept that the stomach and duodenal ulcers may be the result of an infectious agent. They observed that almost 85 to 90 percent of duodenal ulcers and 60 to 80 percent of gastric ulcers had a bacterium in the stomach. This curved bacillus, known as *Helicobacter pylori*, has been known to be present in the stomach for the last one hundred years, but no one paid any attention to this finding until Marshall's work. Now the medical establishment has recognized that *H. pylori* is intimately involved in the causation of these ulcers and is responsive to antibiotics. *H. pylori* is a stubborn organism and a large amount of various antibiotic programs are currently being used and studied for their effectiveness against this organism. These include amoxycillin, tetracycline, metronidazole, bioxin, as well as preparations of bismuth (in the U.S. Pepto-Bismol), and Prilosec®, for periods of two to four weeks with varying degrees of success. Relapses and reinfection do occur, but we still know comparatively little regarding the organism's life cycle, and the development of side effects of some of these antibiotics makes clinical choices still a difficult problem.

Incidentally, to make the problem much more difficult, fragments of the evidence at present suggest that *H. pylori* may play a part in the development of cancer of the stomach. Once antimicrobial agents have gotten rid of the bacteria, they can prevent the recurrence of ulcers throughout the life of the patient, so the old adage, "Once an ulcer, always an ulcer," no longer holds true.

But *H. pylori* may not be the sole factor. The nonsteroidal drugs can cause ulcers without *H. pylori*. As we grow older, more and more of our stomachs contain this bacterium and yet we don't all come down with ulcers. Acid still seems to play a significant part. But *H. pylori* and acid work together, and how each plays its part remains as yet unknown. A whole army of investigators are currently hot on the trail of this culprit and how acid fits into this puzzle.

A Dietary Approach to Peptic Ulcer

We are all aware of the cliché that it's not what you eat, but it's what's eating you, though it is very hard to prove that diet can cause a peptic ulcer and it is most unlikely that diet will cure one. You cannot help thinking that diet can make some difference in the healing of your ulcer, and I share your instinct even if we can't prove it. Before your ulcer was firmly diagnosed, you probably tried to avoid highly seasoned or spicy foods, though you ordinarily enjoyed them.

In the absence of clear-cut scientific proof, it seems prudent to behave rationally. All agree that we should eat a well-balanced and nutritionally adequate diet, but beyond this, what else can one accept as reasonable? Avoiding highly acetic acidic foods and drinks is firmly indicated if acid plays any role in ulcer pain, which we all agree it does to some degree. Indeed, most ulcer sufferers come to this conclusion themselves and have already cut out citrus fruits before they seek treatment. These fruits contain ascorbic acid (vitamin C) and acetic acid. It would certainly be wise to avoid vinegar or dressings containing vinegar. *Bland* is a rather vague word, but it captures the need for a diet that is palatable enough to be eaten while not too appetizing to stimulate the gastric juices excessively.

Remember, this is not a life sentence but a reasonable approach to hasten healing.

Proteins are *amphoteric*—that is, they bind acids and alkali. On the other hand, the products of their digestion, amino acids, stimulate stomach secretion as well so a diet moderately high in protein (fish, chicken, beef, and egg whites) is probably in order.

Fiber—that is, the fiber of vegetables, salads, or fruit—raises a question mark for most individuals. Surely, our patients ask us, "With a sore in the stomach, won't fibrous foods cause injury or at least slow down healing?" The answer seems to be that there is no good evidence that this is so. I encourage my patients to add some moderate amounts of roughage, especially steamed vegetables, canned or cooked fruit, including a banana, and don't insist on their eating salads or raw vegetables.

Fats and oils slow down and cut off acid secretion so why not concentrate on them? Unfortunately, their full effect on blood cholesterol, the high LDLs (the "bad" cholesterol), and the long-term effects on the heart are still the main reasons to avoid foods with a high-fat content, which most Americans still enjoy eating.

Milk has been relied on by most laypersons as the ideal food for ulcers. Milk by its volume, as well as chemical content, can indeed dilute and neutralize acid. Certainly low-fat—that is, 1 to 2 percent milk—will certainly avoid the possibility of too high a fat content in your diet. In the presence of normal kidneys, the high calcium content of milk products is perfectly safe, but I see no special virtue in a high-milk intake for ulcer patients.

By cutting out citrus fruits and juices, we run the risk of reducing our vitamin C intake. But scurvy is not a real risk in most patients' ulcer diets and can be prevented by a small amount of vitamin C in tablet form that can leave the stomach quickly with a glass of water.

So, in the end, we can add very little to the belief that diet does play a major role in ulcer causation or healing. Obviously, having an ulcer does not have any effect on any known food intolerance that we have had in the past. We should still behave in keeping with any past dietary experience, ulcer or not. Since we know that food can act as an antacid and give relief from pain, it follows that we should not skip meals or delay eating too long between meals. Since stretching the wall of the stomach stimulates acid secretion, it is reasonable to have more frequent small meals than one large meal each day.

What Do We Really Know about Foodstuffs and Acid Secretion?

You may very well think I have been walking around the subject of diet and peptic ulcers. Surely, you may ask, have not researchers studied the effect of actual foodstuffs in the process of stimulating acid secretion?

This is a difficult job with humans, but it may be helpful and interesting to see how an animal's stomach, quite similar to ours, responds. Dogs are ideal animals for this type of research, at least in trying to determine the exact response to given foodstuffs. Dr. Charles F. Code and his coworkers at the Mayo Clinic some thirty years ago measured the acid response of about twenty-four foods in a specially prepared dog's stomach. They found that most gastric juices formed within the first hour to hour-and-a-half in most cases, but milk seemed to reach its peak of stimulation in a two to two-and-a-half-hour period after being drunk. Each food group has its own characteristic response; and similar patterns occurred within several distinct groups, such as breads and cheeses, fruits and vegetables, milk and dairy products, and proteins. Protein produced the most acid. Starches, sugar, and fats produced the least.

As a group, meat, fish, and dairy products—the proteins— had the highest acid response, while green peas, oatmeal, french fried potatoes, and some dry cereals the lowest. The foods producing the least amount per 100 calories of substance were fruits, either raw or in juice form, preserved or fresh, butter, white bread, and dry cereals (cornflakes, for example).

This tells us what mostly happens in the process of acid secretion, but this explanation is somewhat artificial. After all, the foods themselves interact in the subject's stomach to create the acids. The complex environment of the stomach thus escapes clear observation.

What about the Three Other Substances We Put in Our Mouths—Caffeine, Alcohol, and Tobacco?

Caffeine is a very strong stimulant of stomach acid so caffeine-containing beverages and foods must also be avoided. Coffee, tea, and cola drinks contain caffeine. So do over-the-counter headache pills and pills we take to keep us from being drowsy. Actually, the list of such sources is quite long (Table 7). In our society, we have become accustomed to large doses of caffeine, and I make no rules forbidding caffeine in healthy individuals. But if you have an ulcer problem, caffeine is out of the question.

While we are on the subject of caffeine, it might be appropriate to recognize that investigators for the first time have shown that caffeine is addictive. Probably the world's most widely used mind-altering drug, caffeine is used by 80 percent of adults in this country, who consume about 280 milligrams of caffeine a day, a little more than the amount of caffeine contained in two cups of coffee. The definition of dependence used in recent studies included withdrawal symptoms, development of increasing tolerance to its effects, the use of caffeine despite aggravation of mental or medical problems, and repeated unsuccessful attempts at stopping. However, in this context, only a small but unknown percentage of Americans are really true caffeine addicts. The addicted consume widely amounts of caffeine; no single level of caffeine intake makes the definition of addiction more likely. Coffee, tea, and cola drinkers all can fit

Table 7. Caffeine Content of Several Common Sources

Substance	Caffeine (in milligrams)
Coca-Cola (12 oz.)	46
Pepsi-Cola (12 oz.)	38
No-Doz®	100
Anacin® (1 tablet)	32
Excedrin® (1 tablet)	65
Decaffeinated coffee (6 oz.)	1–4
Percolated coffee (6 oz.)	40–175
Drip brewed coffee (6 oz.)	60–130
Instant coffee (6 oz.)	25–120
Brewed tea (6 oz.)	20–110
Instant tea (6 oz.)	25–50
Cocoa (6 oz.)	10–25
Milk chocolate (1 oz.)	5
Bittersweet chocolate (1 oz.)	5–10

the addictive pattern. The net effect of current as yet incomplete studies suggest that it is more difficult to give up coffee than most individuals think. The advice the experts give us is to taper off slowly.

Alcohol is not a strong stimulant of stomach acid. Yet you would not poor alcohol over a raw wound or ulceration without wincing. Alcohol can irritate damaged tissues directly, since it passes over areas that are injured by your ulcer. I see no place even for an occasional social drink in the person who suffers from an active ulcer.

Now I will be dogmatic. *Smoking*, especially cigarette smoking, interferes with ulcer healing possibly by interfering with blood flow. The fact is rock solid. You must stop smoking if you wish your ulcer to heal and to stay healed. We all know the important reasons for not smoking, from avoiding cancer of the lung to protecting yourself against heart disease. In most aspects I am a permissive parent, but I will not negotiate with you on the question of smoking. You must stop cold turkey or by using the new nicotine patches, Smoke-Enders®, or hypnosis, or by whatever means you wish or can, but you must stop.

Bland Diets

Traditionally, bland diets have been presented for ulcer patients on the basis that the diet should be palatable enough to be eaten while not too stimulating of the gastric juices of the stomach. But, as I have said, no dietary approach has managed to prevent relapses or recurrences of gastric or duodenal ulcers.

Yet instinctively we feel we want to eat some kinds of food that are "comforting" to the upper GI tract. So we doctors suggest cooked cereals for breakfast with occasional soft boiled eggs, or lightly scrambled eggs in a Teflon pan; lunch of simple chicken or turkey or some fish sandwiches with decaffeinated tea or coffee; dinners of steamed vegetables, rice, potato or pasta, chicken, fish, turkey, red meat or beef, all broiled (avoiding fried foods), canned or cooked fruits, gelatin and simple pudding desserts.

Patients have usually discovered for themselves that citrus fruits (orange, lemon, grapefruit) are poorly tolerated and have traditionally avoided "spicy foods" or highly seasoned ones. Avoidance of alcohol, smoking, and caffeine in any form will pay off in prompter relief of symptoms with possibly less recurrence. Diets of the past have not been able to minimize relapses and recurrences of ulcer symptoms and disease. But studies in the future will define the approach to *H. pylori* more clearly, and we already know that the elimination of *H. pylori* promises eliminating the recurrence of ulcers. Avoiding the nonsteroidal anti-inflammatory drugs (NSAIDs), which include aspirin and varieties of ibuprofen (Advil® and Motrin®), is important, especially in long-term use for conditions like chronic arthritis.

Interestingly, fiber has not been dropped from the diet of ulcer patients, even in the presence of a gastric ulcer, since mechanical factors seem to play little role in slowing healing.

Non-Ulcer Dyspepsia—Indigestion Without a Name

Very often we complain to our physician, "I am having trouble with my stomach." We point to the upper part of the abdomen where we experience discomfort that verges on pain. We often have a slight sense of nausea, but rarely do we vomit. We have no trouble swallowing, but are uncomfortable near the end of a meal or directly after finishing it. We feel bloated and distended, and we experience more than the usual sense of fullness.

Doctors label these symptoms of indigestion as *dyspepsia*, and like the patient, they seem to be sure that these symptoms do not arise from organic disease of the upper gastrointestinal tract, gallbladder, or pancreas. Patients and doctors are reassured and pleased when the necessary tests are performed and eliminate organic disease, but the discomfort still persists.

What help can our dietary recommendations give those suffering from dyspepsia, a condition affecting countless individuals?

One thing is certain—in some individuals, these dyspeptic symptoms overlap and are part of an irritable bowel syndrome, probably the most common reason patients seek out gastrointestinal specialists. The heart of the problems in the irritable bowel syndrome is on the lower gastrointestinal tract, and here, too, no organic disorder accounts for its cause. I will deal with and discuss the role of diet in the irritable bowel syndrome in detail later in this book. However, once you learn that your upper intestinal sense of indigestion is labeled *non-ulcerative dyspepsia*, you realize that this problem is not an easy one to treat. It seems a wastebasket diagnosis, a label put to a pattern that is not well understood, but involves no organic disease. This is true enough. Your physician will need to try to sort out the different pattern of your specific complaints, so the particular torments you suffer can be eliminated.

One set of dyspeptic symptoms seems to resemble those produced by reflux, in which the acid contents of the stomach enter the esophagus. A second pattern of dyspepsia suggests the symptoms of a peptic ulcer. A third set of symptoms suggests distention of the stomach due to air swallowing (aerophagia). Yet a fourth type of dyspepsia lumps a group of patients who have the symptoms of fullness, burping, or belching, along with an inability to finish a meal of normal size. These patients seem to be telling us that they are having trouble emptying the stomach in a normal fashion. They appear to have a motor problem, a problem of moving food and fluid along from the stomach into the upper small bowel. Doctors label it a *motility* problem. Even if we don't know the exact cause of these different types of non-ulcerative dyspepsia, our physicians need to try to answer our questions and relieve our discomfort.

1. Those with symptoms that resemble reflux should turn to the advice I offer in this chapter in the section on "Heartburn and Peptic Esophagitis." While this may seem tedious, these guidelines may offer relief.
2. Those whose dyspepsia mimics ulcer disease, although tests fail to reveal an ulcer, should follow the restrictions I have outlined on pages 58–62 which cover peptic ulcer disease.
3. Those who suffer from air swallowing are easy to help in theory but difficult in practice. These are the individuals who suck on a pipe all day, even if they do not light the tobacco. Others keep a real or fake cigarette in their mouth and are never going to stop cigarette smoking. They also include folks who gulp down their breakfast and lunch quickly in order to save time, avoid being late for important meetings or their regular train schedule. This group also consumes carbonated beverages with all their meals, which add to the gases in the stomach and upper gastrointestinal tract. Very often they are the ones who are eating and talking vociferously at the same time. Long-

standing habits of eating and drinking are not easily corrected, even with all the will in the world. Air swallowers need to follow the general healthy diet I have described in Chapter 3 and need to take time for meals, skip the carbonated beverages, stop smoking, and stop eating and talking at the same time. They may need biofeedback methods to help them learn healthy eating habits or to quit smoking.

4. If your difficulties seem to arise from failure of the stomach to move its contents during and after a meal, this can be tested using a gastric-emptying scan. The problem here is not in the chemistry of the food, nor in its fiber content, the indigestible portion of foods, but in the pumping action of the stomach muscles. In addition to the dietary points I have already made in this book regarding the elements of a well-balanced, high-fiber, high-carbohydrate, low-fat diet, I would stress here the fact that fats tend to slow down even the normal emptying of the stomach, so I would advise those suffering from a motility problem to reduce their fat intake significantly. It will be good for their hearts and blood vessels, as well as their stomachs. Important new drugs that stimulate the stomach to empty more effectively are now available, and you will need your doctor's advice regarding their usage. They include one called Cispride, now known commercially as Propulsid®, and, interestingly enough, the antibiotic erythromycin may at times also work as well.

What about H. pylori and Non-Ulcer Dyspepsia?

Infestation of the stomach with *H. pylori* increases as we grow older and does not seem to play a significant role in non-ulcer dyspepsia. However, if any of the current tests—endoscopic biopsy, blood antibodies, or breath tests for *H. pylori* overgrowth in the stomach—confirm that it is present, I think it might be worthwhile to try antibiotics to see if they make any difference. My experience thus far has been far from clear-cut. Of the many trials using this approach that have been published, about half

the patients seem to show improvement, and yet we really don't
know if this is because of chance or a placebo response. *H. pylori* is a stubborn organism to get rid of, and the antibiotics used
at present require two to three weeks of medication; some drugs
obviously will create side effects in sensitive individuals.

Since *H. pylori* may result in future stomach or duodenal
ulcers, has been implicated in the development of gastric cancer, and may be important in some localized stomach lympho-
mas, I make every effort to eliminate this "boarder" in the
patient's stomach without promising the individual that it will
eliminate the non-ulcer dyspepsia.

5
✳ ✳ ✳

THE GALLBLADDER
IN THE
MODERN AGE

The upper intestinal tract is so well programmed that bile
enters the duodenum just at the time it is needed to help
digest the fats of our diet. Since the liver is manufacturing bile
all the time, this exact timing is carried out by the gallbladder,
which is the receptacle for the temporary storage of bile. When
the fats in the diet enter the duodenum, they release the hormone known as *cholecystokinin* that causes the gallbladder to
contract and empty its bile content just at the time and place
where it is needed to facilitate the next step of fat digestion.
Fats consist of long chains of fatty acids that are attached to
glycerol; these are known as the *triglycerides*. These fatty substances do not dissolve in water; as we all know, oil and water
do not mix. To be absorbed, the triglycerides undergo a complex
chemical rearrangement. The triglyceride is split into small
components, the fatty acids, by the pancreatic fat-splitting enzymes, the lipases, and the particles are then enclosed in bile
salts secreted in the liver bile. The reorganized particles are

called *micelles*, and these can now be transported across the lining cells in the intestine and thus be absorbed. The main problem associated with the gallbladder when things go wrong is that it can produce stones, which can cause serious difficulties and episodes of pain.

What about the Things the Gallbladder Is Blamed for?

The gallbladder is blamed unfairly for any discomfort in the right upper portion of the abdomen whenever there may be burping, bloating, or belching, or whenever there is any indigestion at all connected with fatty foods. This is understandable since gallstones and disease of the gallbladder are so common. It is estimated that between 10 and 20 percent of the world's population has stones. A recent estimate suggested the majority of individuals above sixty years of age have gallstones as well.

Who Is Likely to Get Gallstones?

In approaching the problem of preventing gallstones, we must first consider who is most at risk. First, there are some families who have the genetic predisposition to form stones. The Pima Indians in southwestern United States, for example, have a very high incidence: 85 to 90 percent of the women and 70 to 80 percent of the men are affected with gallstones.

Women are more likely than men to have stones and this susceptibility increases with each pregnancy. While young people can develop stones, the incidence of gallstones increases with age, especially as we approach middle age. Those that are overweight suffer more. It is important to know that the obese individual who attempts to drop pounds by trying a crash diet can precipitate stones in the gallbladder. While one might suppose that individuals with higher levels of cholesterol in their blood or bile will have more cholesterol stones, this is not the case. However, some individuals with unusually high levels of triglycerides in the blood do have a greater chance of forming stones. The older forms of contraceptive pills with high estrogen levels seem to have played a part in the problem of stone formation, but this is rarely seen nowadays with the improved low-estrogen pill.

What Causes Gallstones?

About 70 percent of stones are *cholesterol stones*. The other type of gallbladder stone is the *pigment stone* found when the bile contains excessive amounts of bilirubin, the breakdown product of hemoglobin, which is an element of red blood cells. The pigment stones form in the individual whose red blood cells are destroyed more rapidly than normal. This includes individuals suffering from chronic hemolytic anemia, sickle cell disease, or malaria.

The cholesterol stones result from a defect in the liver that forms an abnormal bile. This bile is oversaturated with cholesterol and undersaturated with bile acid, which dissolves bile cholesterol. The stones are formed from this imbalance of overproduction of cholesterol by the liver and the concomitant undersecretion of bile acids.

But Surely One Needs to Have Trouble in the Gallbladder Itself?

Irregular meal patterns may lead to longer storage time for bile in the gallbladder, in some individuals, but this does not necessarily lead to stones. Infection in the gallbladder wall does interfere with that organ's ability to absorb cholesterol and thus reduce its supersaturation. Finally, bile is recycled by mechanisms in the ileum. The bile salt pool can be reduced by disease or by surgical removal of parts of the ileum, as in Crohn's disease.

How Can Dietary Manipulation or Changes in
Eating Habits Prevent or Treat Gallstones or
Disease of the Gallbladder?

For those without stones, more regular eating patterns without skipping meals will prevent too long a period of storage of bile in the gallbladder. Reduction of triglycerides in the blood seems the rational thing to do, and some would favor the idea of a high-fiber, low-fat diet.

Many individuals have been discovered by accident in the course of other investigations to have asymptomatic gallstones of the cholesterol variety—stones that are silent and produce no discomfort. For these individuals, it may be prudent to avoid obesity and to reduce any overweight by very small steps over a long period of time, to avoid a rapid weight loss that can very easily precipitate attacks of gallstones. Rapid weight loss may precipitate gallstones by mobilizing large amounts of cholesterol from the fat deposits of the body.

For those whose stones have been discovered because of episodes of *biliary colic*, which is an attack of severe right upper abdominal pain due to a stone or stones attempting to get out of the gallbladder, there is now a medical program that will help dissolve these stones.

For those with cholesterol stones, especially small stones, the bile salts have been in use for a long time. Chenodeoxycholic acid (CDCA) and more recently ursodecolic acid (UDCA), or a combination of these two, may dissolve about 23 percent of stones. But with the presence of the gallbladder, there is a tendency for these stones to reform. In fact, about one-third of stones will reappear within three and a half years to seven years. This method of bile salts dissolving cholesterol stones probably has a limited role to play in those too sick for the conventional or the newer forms of laparoscopic-assisted cholecystectomy. In this procedure, the surgeon views the interior of the abdomen through videoscopic cameras and removes the gallbladder through a very small abdominal incision. The result is a more rapid recovery and a shorter hospital stay.

For those with stones who have suffered at least one episode of gallbladder colic and elect to continue to live with their stones, it would be prudent to reduce the fat intake of the diet, not to dissolve the stones, but instead to prevent a fatty meal from releasing large amounts of cholecystokinin, stimulating the gallbladder to contract vigorously and thus precipitate a colic attack. While this appears prudent and I think rational, it has never been proven scientifically. I have observed many patients who have had only one episode of colic and have never had another that the patient ascribes to improved eating habits, especially the reduction of fat intake. It is impossible for the normal individual to reduce the intake of fat so much so the gallbladder fails to contract at all. The gallbladder, after all, plays an important role in breaking down fat in the diet—fat which seems a mainstay in the American diet.

A Dietary Approach to Gallstones and Gallbladder Disease

The advice we can offer individuals with these problems is indeed quite limited—avoid obesity, avoid drastic crash diets, follow regular eating patterns, and avoid skipping food for long periods of time.

We should hold the gallbladder responsible only for severe attacks of biliary colic, not for every episode of indigestion following a fatty meal or for every burp or belch. If you have stones, no diet at present will dissolve them or correct the imbalance between the cholesterol and the bile salts. Reducing the fat content of your diet is worthwhile in itself and may reduce the triggering effect of fat that releases the hormone cholecystokinin to the gallbladder and that leads to the problems we have looked at in this chapter.

6

* * *

DIET AND DISORDERS
OF THE PANCREAS

The pancreas is an important gland in the digestive process and pours its external secretions, the pancreatic juice, into the upper duodenum. The enzymes of this fluid digest fat, protein, and starch into smaller units, a vital step in the digestion and absorption of our foodstuffs and a crucial one in the digestion of fats. The pancreas works in conjunction with the bile salts of the liver, which, as we learned in the previous chapter, are stored in the gallbladder and liberated into the duodenum at just the right time to meet up with pancreatic lipase—the fat-splitting enzyme.

The pancreas can malfunction acutely—in what we call *acute pancreatitis*—or it can slowly and chronically go awry, taking a chronic form we call *chronic pancreatitis*, or the pancreas can develop benign or malignant tumors. Since the pancreas also secretes insulin into the bloodstream to regulate our sugar metabolism, acute or chronic forms of pancreatitis or tumor formation will disturb this metabolism and present a clinical picture of insulin-dependent diabetes in the adult. The inherited disorder of the very young, cystic fibrosis, also can result in the insufficient external secretions of the pancreatic gland, resembling chronic pancreatitis.

By far the most common causes of pancreatitis in both the chronic and acute forms are alcohol and biliary tract disease. Next in importance is the genetic disorder, cystic fibrosis, which may involve the pancreas. Especially intriguing is the long list of *drugs* that cause pancreatitis. They include diuretics (water pills), such as chlorothiazide (Diuril®), furosemide (Lasix®), antibiotics such as sulfonamides, salazopyrine (Azulfidine®), and tetracycline. Immunosuppressant drugs such as azathioprine, or 6-mercaptopurine, as well as anti-tumor drugs such as vincristine, can also induce pancreatitis. Still, from a statistical point of view, alcohol and biliary tract disease are the main culprits.

What Can We Do about Preventing Pancreatitis?

Alcohol is still the most likely cause of pancreatitis in the Westernized world. There is no question that avoiding alcohol in our daily diet will markedly reduce the chances of getting pancreatitis, both in the acute and chronic forms. There are many good health reasons to limit alcohol intake to no more than a glass of wine, or 1 or 2 ounces of spirits, daily, which I have already discussed in Chapter 3. Since alcohol is not necessary for body nutrition, one need not drink at all. Individuals who consider themselves mild to moderate social drinkers often precipitate their attacks of pancreatitis by combining several cocktails before dinner, with wine during the meal, and then ordering a very fatty meal. I have already emphasized, maybe overemphasized, the need to reduce total fat in our American diet. This common dining out scenario should be avoided. Certainly, if you have had any attacks of pancreatitis or a precipitating incident, alcohol should be a no-no, as well as avoiding a rich, fatty meal.

The continued abusive use of alcohol is without a doubt the chief cause of chronic pancreatitis. There is little hope in preventing the inexorable damage to the pancreas; the scarring of tissue and insufficiency of the pancreatic enzymes lead to chronic pain (sometimes needing powerful narcotics) that leads to weight loss, diarrhea, and the wasting of muscle mass. There is no escape from this chain of events, and strict avoidance of any and all forms of alcohol is essential.

How gallbladder disease, especially gallstones, causes pancreatitis is far from clear despite fifty years of research. But some facts are clear. In both women as well as men, gallstones are associated with recurrent attacks of pancreatitis. In the previous chapter on the gallbladder, I have outlined what little we know about avoiding gallstones. Yet several guidelines can help. Try to eat three meals daily at regular intervals without going for too long without meals, don't skip meals, and reduce the triglyceride level in your bloodstream by following a high-fiber, low-fat diet. Avoid crash diets. Rapid weight loss followed by repeated regaining will increase the risk of gallstones and pancreatitis. If you are known to have gallstones, it is obviously wise to avoid alcohol and a fatty diet, which may trigger an acute episode of pancreatitis.

Should Gallbladders with Stones Be Removed to Prevent the Development of Pancreatitis?

This question nowadays is of more than academic interest since the new laparoscopic-assisted form of gallbladder removal has made such a procedure far easier for the patient than the surgical procedures of the past, has shortened the hospital stay, and has reduced the postoperative discomfort and pain. Just having one attack of gallbladder colic, however, does not mean it is necessary to remove the gallbladder, except under special circumstances (the young woman with many small stones who is contemplating further pregnancies). Moreover, not every attack of biliary colic is attended by a concomitant attack of pancreatitis. I certainly advise no alcohol and a high-fiber, low-fat diet to minimize the chances of pancreatitis.

But documented evidence of pancreatitis in an individual with biliary stones following an attack of gallbladder colic certainly makes removal of the gallbladder a reasonable move to avoid further problems.

A Dietary Approach to Chronic Pancreatitis

The pancreas has great regenerative power, and the gland can and does recover functionally after one episode of pancreatitis. The problem arises if there is a persistence of distress resulting from pancreatic disease after the triggering mechanism has been removed (cessation of long-standing alcohol abuse or cure of long-standing undiagnosed gallbladder disease). Here dietary adjustment is probably the only method we have of helping this serious and disturbing situation. We must replace the missing pancreatic enzymes with one of the many available forms of pancreatic extracts that contain amylase (which splits starch), lipase (which splits fat), and trypsin (which splits proteins). Patients with insufficient pancreatic secretions seem to handle starch and protein fairly well. Their main difficulty is in digesting fat, which is so important for caloric intake and weight gain or maintenance. It is not necessary for the individual to reduce the fat intake to zero, which indeed cannot be accomplished, but to take moderate amounts of fat and to supply the upper intestine with adequate amounts of pancreatic enzyme replacements. These replacement enzymes are first taken at the beginning, during, and at the end of each meal, accompanying the food, and along with each and every snack. Since the enzyme preparations are taken by mouth, they run the inevitable risk of being digested and partially destroyed by the digestive juices of the stomach. So these persons must also take some of the histamine II acid-blocking agents (Tagamet®, Zantac®, Axid®, or Pepcid®) well before each meal to minimize the destruction of the enzyme preparation in the stomach. With this program in place, we can then begin to increase the fat intake slowly up to the desired 30 percent level, increasing the pancreatic enzyme replacement as needed to take care of any increased amount of fat to be digested.

If this approach does not work, or the patient is intolerant of the fat load, then there are other forms of fat that can be given by mouth. These are the medium-chain triglycerides (MCTs), which do not need the bile salt–lipase treatment to be absorbed. The oil itself (MCT) can be taken directly, by mouth as a liquid, or can be used in cooking. It has a high caloric value and aids in weight gain. Many of us will have memories of the cod liver oil their parents gave them as children; this preparation is not unlike that in consistency and not unpleasant in taste.

7

* * *

MALABSORPTION: STARVATION IN THE MIDST OF PLENTY

The most dramatic form of malabsorption is celiac disease, often called *celiac sprue* or nontropical sprue, and more recently, *gluten enteropathy.*

First appearing in young children, this disease can flare up in adulthood or even appear later in life. The clinical picture is a dramatic one—weakness, weight loss, diarrhea and bloating, distention and cramping, muscle wasting, fatigue, and loss of energy. These symptoms can all be explained by the failure of the intestine to absorb calories, especially fat calories, and minerals such as iron and calcium, which is associated with a slow protein leak in the intestine from the blood. There is often an accompanying swelling of the ankles together with failure to absorb the fat-soluble vitamins A, D, and K. All this malfunctioning follows from an abnormality of the lining cells of the small intestine, the loss of the microscopic elements of the villi that are essential to intestinal absorption.

Yet all these symptoms can disappear and the patient can

make a complete turnaround simply by adhering to a strict diet. What is amazing is that this disorder, known for two millennia, responds to withdrawal in the diet of the wheat protein gluten, which is also present in other grains and cereals. The disease was well known and well described by Galen about 250 A.D. and carefully studied in the middle of the nineteenth century by very observant physicians who suspected that the error in nontropical sprue lay in the diet of these unfortunate individuals. The modern era, a triumphant one in gastroenterology, is essentially indebted to the work of Willem-Karo Dicke (1905–1962), a brilliant Dutch pediatrician. As early as 1934 and 1936, Dicke had started experiments with wheat-free diets in celiac children. His experience in World War II, when the delivery of bread to his young patients in hospitals was reduced by the war, persuaded him further that merely eating less cereals and wheat improved the clinical condition of his patients. His thesis in 1950 was entitled "Celiac Disease: Investigation of Harmful Effects of Certain Types of Cereal on Patients with Celiac Disease," and was published by The University of Utrecht, The Netherlands. It became a classic. Workers soon showed that it was the gluten fraction in these foods that was at fault, and further refinements led to the discovery that it was the *gliadin* fraction of the gluten that was the chief culprit.

Genetic factors are probably involved and some postulate a specific infection as triggering the syndrome, whereas others postulate some defect in the mechanism of the intestinal lining cells as being at fault. But two facts remain uncontroverted— once a celiac, always a celiac, and gluten withdrawal is the cure. The intestinal cells will repair their villi if treatment is instituted. Curiously enough, a skin condition, *dermatitis herpetiformis*, Dühring's disease, is related to celiac disease. In this disorder of gluten sensitivity, skin manifestations are predominant, with intestinal difficulty less obvious. Many of its sufferers have asymptomatic intestinal disease, as do some of their relatives. The skin reaction usually responds to gluten withdrawal from the diet.

Dietary Treatment of Celiac Sprue

The cure seems simple enough. Avoid gluten that is found in certain grains—wheat, barley, rye, oats, millet, and buckwheat. But following such a diet in real life is complex. If you or your child has gluten enteropathy, it poses further problems when serving meals to the whole family and when eating out in restaurants. It requires scrupulous reading of food labels when considering prepared foods, not always easy to do. But there is no risk in a diet free of gluten; gluten is not essential as a protein and its amino acid components are replaced by other foods. There are many possible benefits from following the gluten-free diet, and the diet is a good one. One does not require drugs with their side effects, but strict adherence is required. Sufferers feel better quite quickly; however, the intestine requires three to six months to restore itself to normality.

A General List of Foods Allowed and Foods to Avoid

The following list (Table 8) is based on the publications of the Celiac Sprue Association, United States of America, Inc. (CSA/USA), which has played an important part in the entire concept of self-help for patients with this disorder. The interesting and important publications of this group were obtained from the association's headquarters: P.O. Box 31700, Omaha, Nebraska 68131–0700, telephone: (402) 558–0600. Wheat, barley, rye and oats contain the gliadin fraction of gluten which is the culprit in this disorder. It is estimated that about 40 percent of new patients also react unfavorably to millet, soy, and buckwheat, so these too should be eliminated from the diet.

Further dietary information can be obtained from the American Celiac Society Dietary Support Coalition, 58 Musano Court, West Orange, New Jersey 07052–4114.

Table 8. Diet for Celiac Sprue

Wheat, barley, rye, and oats contain the gliadin fraction that is harmful to persons with celiac sprue (also known as *gluten-sensitive enteropathy*. About 40 percent of newly diagnosed celiacs also react unfavorably to millet, soy, and buckwheat. As a general guideline, these grains should also be avoided.

	Foods Allowed	Foods to Avoid
1. Grains	Rice, corn, and most persons do well on soybeans; arrowroot is also allowed.	Wheat, barley, rye, oats, and probably millet and buckwheat for most people. Be careful of breads and ricecakes that often contain both rye and millet. Avoid wheat starch; the manufacturers say it does contain small amounts of gluten; when questioned, it is represented as 92 to 97 percent glutenfree. Many communion wafers may also be made of wheat starch.
2. Vegetables	Use fresh, frozen, dried, or canned unless they contain thickening agents. For example, flour is used in most canned peas. In canned products, avoid emulsifiers, preservatives, stabilizers, and food starch unless its source is known.	Read INGREDIENT labels.

(continued)

	Foods Allowed	Foods to Avoid
3. Fruits	Fruits are simpler. Use most fresh, frozen, dried, or canned fruits. A few contain additives or preservatives. Read labels.	Avoid thickening agents for some fruits and pie fillings.
4. Meats	Use fresh, frozen, and canned meats.	Avoid luncheon meats, prepared sausages, canned meats with preservatives, cereals, flour, food starch, and grains.
5. Breads	Use rice flours, white or brown, arrowroot, potato, and tapioca. Use soybean (soya) if tolerated; add pea, corn, or bean flours for variety.	Avoid low-gluten flours and wheat starch; flours with wheat, barley, rye, and oats; soybean (soya) if sensitive to it; millet and buckwheat.
6. Cereals	Hot cereals made from cornmeal, cream of rice, hominy, rice, cold cereals such as puffed rice, Kellogg's Sugar Pops, Post's Fruity and Chocolate Pebbles, Van Brode's cornflakes and crisp rice, General Mill's Coca Puffs (unless sensitive to chocolate).	Avoid cereals with wheat, barley, rye, oats, millet, and buckwheat. Avoid bran, graham, wheat germ, and bulgur. Do not use the several cereals available that contain malt unless approved by your physician.

(continued)

	Foods Allowed	Foods to Avoid
7. Cheeses	All aged hard cheeses such as cheddar, swiss, edam, and parmesan. Check ingredient list on cottage cheese, cream cheese, and all pasteurized, processed cheese. Avoid cheeses with vegetable gum and preservatives.	Avoid all cheese foods, cheese spreads, and nondairy products in the dairy counter such as spreads and the chip n' dip mixes.
8. Salad Dressings	Start with the several Kraft dressings which are gluten-free or make your own. Read labels before each purchase. The ingredients may change with each batch number. Be aware of the use of grain vinegar.	Several commercial salad dressings contain one or more of the offending grains, preservatives, food starch, emulsifiers, stabilizers, or dyes. Avoid the product unless contents are known. Avoid products with secondary foods added. For example, tomato soup, in some form, contains wheat flour.

(continued)

Table 8. Diet for Celiac Sprue (continued)

	Foods Allowed	Foods to Avoid
9. Drinks and Juices	Fresh brewed coffee other than a ground coffee with grain added. For example, Mellow Roast. Tea, chocolate made with cocoa, fruit juices, carbonated drinks. Avoid most of the instant drinks which are processed with or have additives, stabilizers, or emulsifiers added. For example, Hawaiian Punch. Only a few root beers allowed.	Omit all instant coffees, instant tea, instant cocoa mixed, Postum, Ovaltine, malted milk, commercial chocolate milk which may have cereal added, and ground coffees which contain grain and some root beers. Know the product, read labels, look for excipients (stuffers).
10. Flours	Arrowroot starch, corn flour, cornmeal, corn starch, potato flour, potato starch, rice bran, rice flour, rice polish, soy flour, tapioca flour, tapioca starch.	All flours containing wheat, barley, rye, oats, millet, or buckwheat; also avoid wheat starch, triticale, and amaranth.
11. Soups	Homemade broth with allowed ingredients.	Most canned soups and soup mixes, especially bouillon in powder, cubes, or canned form.

	Foods Allowed	Foods to Avoid
12. Fats and Oils	Most celiacs do best on corn oils; most corn oils, margarines, butter, lard, cream, pure mayonnaise, peanut butters, and most hydrogenated vegetable oils are acceptable. Some margarines have flour as an additive. Start with Fleischmanns.	Check out vegetable oils for additives and margarines for possible offenders before using. Look for salad dressings which contain gluten-free stabilizers. Read labels.
13. Vinegars	Use apple cider and wine vinegars.	Avoid distilled white vinegar which uses a grain mash as a starting material.
14. Alcoholic Beverages	Wine and brandies without preservatives and added dyes; most celiacs do best on white wines; potato vodka, not grain vodka; most rums and tequila are okay.	Avoid all beers, ales, and anything made from grain alcohol; all whiskey, bourbons, Canadian blends; most liqueurs; corn whiskey also since it uses a grain mash.
15. Soy Sauce	Use those that do not contain wheat or barley (LaChoy).	Most soy sauces do contain gluten, especially Kikkoman. Avoid house soy sauces.

(continued)

Table 8. Diet for Celiac Sprue (continued)

	Foods Allowed	Foods to Avoid
16. Crackers and Snack Foods	Rice wafers; pure cornmeal chips and tortillas; popcorn; selected soya crackers.	All others containing the nonallowed grains or coatings of selected soy sauces. Watch out for "pure corn products" that may be dried on a conveyor belt dusted with wheat flour.
17. Desserts	Custard; junket; homemade puddings from cornstarch, tapioca, and rice; gelatin desserts; selected pudding mixes; ice cream and sherbet if they do not contain wheat flour or gluten stabilizers; products made with allowed flours.	All products prepared with the nonallowed grains; ice cream cones and ice creams which contain gluten stabilizers; most commercially prepared mixes for cakes, cookies, and other desserts.
18. Sweets	Sugar; honey; nonbuttered syrup; molasses; most jellies and jams; plain hard candy; marshmallows; gumdrops and homemade or commercial candies made with allowed ingredients.	Check for commercial candies containing the nonallowed grains and gluten stabilizers.

	Foods Allowed	Foods to Avoid
19. Meats or Meat Substitutes	All meats, fish, poultry, and eggs prepared without the nonallowed grains; bacteria-ripened cheeses and processed cheeses if they do not contain a gluten stabilizer; cottage cheese and cream cheese if the vegetable gum used does not contain a forbidden grain.	Several of the luncheon meats, sausages, and frankfurters may contain a grain as an excipient (stuffer) or as a part of a gluten stabilizer; turkey with HVP injected as a part of basting (avoid self-basting fowl); cheese products containing wheat flour and oat gum.
20. Potato or Pasta Starches	White and sweet potatoes; hams; hominy; rice and wild rice; gluten-free and corn pastas; look for oriental rice noodles or bean noodles.	Regular noodles, spaghetti, macaroni, and most packaged rice mixes. See product ingredient listing for clarification. Watch out for wild rice which has been sprayed with insecticide.
21. Yogurt	Use yogurts without milk added if lactose intolerant. Start with Dannon or Yoplait.	Several yogurts on the market contain both milk and a thickening agent. Know the product before using.

(continued)

Table 8. Diet for Celiac Sprue (continued)

	Foods Allowed	Foods to Avoid
22. Miscellaneous	Salt; pepper; herbs; spices; nuts; coconut; chocolate; pure cocoa; flavorings, if not made with alcohol, choose imitations; monosodium glutamate (MSG); yogurt, if made with allowed ingredients; steak sauce, except for persons with extreme sensitivity.	Some curry powder; most white pepper; some dry seasoning mixes; some gravy mixes and extracts; some meat sauces; some catsup, mustard, and horseradish because of the vinegar; some chewing gum; most dips; vanilla and flavorings made with alcohol.

A Final Word on the Gluten-Free Diet

Do not be overwhelmed by this detailed list. The essence is simple. Wheat, rye, oats, and barley are the chief culprits. For some, add millet, soy, and buckwheat to the list. There are a few rare individuals who are sensitive to chicken and eggs as well. If you stick to the diet, you or your child will do well. While some celiac patients have difficulty with dairy products due to primary lactase deficiency, intolerance of milk and dairy products because they are lactose intolerant, most celiac patients gain tolerance to milk and dairy products in response to a gluten-free diet. Calcium and vitamin D should be added to the diet as well, in tablet supplements, since this will aid those celiac patients who have difficulty with milk products.

Malabsorption in the Case of the Shortened Bowel

Malabsorption can also take place when some areas of the small intestine are lost by disease or shortened by surgical procedures that remove long stretches of the bowel or bypass obstructions created by inflamed, infected, or scarred stenotic bowel. These patients suffer from severe malabsorption of nutrients, and it is customary to increase the fat in a patient's diet in the hope of increasing the amount absorbed, even though some fat may be lost in the stool. But this rarely works.

There are several ways one can attempt to overcome the limited absorption of the *short bowel syndrome* as it is called. One way is to use medium-chain triglycerides (MCTs) as the principal form of fat. Remember, one gram of fat yields 9 calories, whereas one gram of carbohydrate or protein yields only 4 calories. In contrast to long-chain fatty acids in our normal diet, these medium-chain triglycerides do not need to be changed into micelles with the aid of bile salts and pancreatic lipase. They can be absorbed directly without any chemical transformation. This can overcome the handicap of a shortened bowel.

The oil itself (MCT) can be used for cooking, salad dressing, or just taken by the tablespoon, yielding a large number of calories. Mead-Johnson has also prepared another liquid form, Portagen®, which can be taken by mouth and which is absorbed by the bloodstream traveling to the liver. However, Portagen contains lactose and some people may be intolerant of lactose.

Another way of increasing the caloric absorption in individuals fortunate enough to have a normal colon, despite a shortened bowel, is to take advantage of the fact that the colon can absorb carbohydrates, and this may be a crucial factor for saving calories in patients with severe malabsorption. By giving the patient a high-carbohydrate diet—60 percent carbohydrate, 20 percent fat, and 20 percent protein calories—the individual may be able to absorb more calories from the diet than from a high-fat diet. It is believed that the extra dietary carbohydrate is absorbed in the colon after being converted into short-chain fatty acids, the preferred food for the colon. For both normal individuals and those with a shortened bowel, the high-carbohydrate diet takes advantage of the fact that under certain circumstances the colon can digest and absorb some forms of carbohydrate in the form of short-chain fatty acids. Thus the large intestine is important in the digestion of carbohydrates and aids in the salvage of calories in patients with short bowel syndrome and severe malabsorption.

8

* * *

IRRITABLE BOWEL SYNDROME

U nder the umbrella term, *irritable bowel syndrome* (IBS), we lump together a group of symptoms that involve the lower intestinal tract, usually the colon, for which we can find no structural cause after a detailed study. These include

1. Pain relieved by having a bowel movement that may be associated with a change in the frequency and the consistency of the stool.
2. Looser and more frequent bowels with lower abdominal pain.
3. Feelings of a bloated and distended abdomen, or the feeling that your abdomen is swollen.
4. Some mucus in the stool that looks like the uncooked whites of an egg or what you blow out of your nose when you have a cold.
5. Very often the most common sensation you feel is that you have not completely emptied your bowel after a movement

and need to go back to pass another "installment"; this is a sense of "incomplete evacuation," as I have called it.

All these symptoms may alternate with periods of constipation, defined as less than three stools per week, or the need to strain or squeeze 25 percent of the time. The irritable bowel syndrome is the most common reason why patients consult gastroenterologists. Indeed, some think that 40 percent of the practice of gastroenterologists is devoted to the irritable bowel. Quite interestingly, the majority of individuals who have these symptoms do not consult a physician. They accept the irritable bowel syndrome as the cost of contemporary living.

The most arduous part of the management of a patient with the irritable bowel syndrome is the need to exclude organic disease of the gastrointestinal tract, especially the lower small intestine and the colon, so a lot of your doctor's time, your patience, and money are spent undergoing tests that reveal no organic or structural defect. You are reassured by your doctor that your complaint is part of the irritable bowel, and that it has no grave consequences. It will not shorten or alter your life expectancy, nor will it lead to other diseases, but you want and need more assurance than that. You want relief from your symptoms and, above all, information regarding your diet.

While the greatest portion of patients consulting physicians who specialize in the intestinal tract may complain of irritable bowel syndrome, this chapter on the role of diet will be one of the shortest because we know so little about the fundamental nature of the irritable bowel. In the recent past it was assumed that the irritable bowel resulted from disordered motility, the movements or contractions of the intestine. More recently, emphasis has shifted to the fact that there may be increased sensitivity to the sensations arising in the lower bowel in people with the irritable bowel syndrome.

But even before we look at the role of food in this syndrome, we need to review your habits. I believe that even without firm double-blind controlled clinical trials to instruct us, it is a safe assumption that irritants such as tobacco, caffeine, and alcohol contribute to the discomfort of this syndrome and should be stopped—I refer to these as "The Big Three."

Tobacco

There are plenty of compelling reasons for not smoking. If you smoke and suffer from IBS, you should be aware that nicotine can be an irritant. Air swallowed during smoking can also contribute to intestinal gas. Stop smoking, using whatever technique you can find—stopping cold turkey, using Smoke-Enders®, even hypnosis (this last one hasn't worked too well or too often for my patients). To quit cigarette smoking is not easy, even for highly motivated and medically informed patients, including doctors. The nicotine patch along with supportive counseling may help some individuals.

Caffeine

Since caffeine is clearly upsetting to the bowel, a trial of stopping all caffeine-containing beverages and food should be used. You will need to avoid coffee, tea, chocolate, and cola drinks containing caffeine. From a food chemist I learned years ago that discarding the first cup of tea made from a fresh tea bag and drinking tea brewed from the used bag reduces the theobromine and the caffeine of the remaining cup. You will also need to avoid other sources of caffeine in your diet that are not as obvious and are listed in Table 7.

Alcohol

Although I am generally not opposed to "moderate" use of alcohol, I think a trial of stopping alcohol consumption is in order. Many patients find that wine, especially red wine, contributes to their discomfort.

Diet

Food, Milk, and Milk Products

By the time most patients get to see me with their irritable bowel symptoms, they have discovered for themselves whether they can tolerate milk and milk products. If there is any doubt or if I have considered a possible milk intolerance, I suggest a two-week trial of withdrawal of milk and milk products from the diet. Yogurt seems to be tolerated because the organisms in yogurt supply the needed enzyme *lactase*. I have not found that a lactose-tolerance test, similar to a glucose-tolerance test for diabetes, has helped me in this connection, and so I don't subject my patients to this testing. If they are truly lactase-deficient, adding the enzyme lactase to milk may be worthwhile, since preparations of this substance (Lactaid®, for example) are now available. A few of my patients have found that taking Lactaid tablets before eating milk products is helpful.

Fiber

Few people in the Western world have not heard that fiber, bran, and other bulk-forming foods are good for the intestine. As a result, many of us are eating bran muffins, adding bran to our breakfast cereals, or taking some form of plant seed such as Metamucil® at night to avoid constipation, diverticulosis, diverticulitis, and cancer of the colon. But despite this hope that a high-fiber diet will help solve the irritable bowel syndrome, the experience of time and of our patients has been disillusioning. It has been far from proven that lack of fiber is an important factor in all instances of IBS, and not everyone with IBS feels better on a high-fiber or bran diet. Indeed, some, or even many, may feel worse.

On the other hand, if you are among those who have dry, hard, constipated stools, an increase of fiber is clearly in order. The plant seeds tend to bind water and so help in the diarrheal phases of IBS. You may have eliminated salads and fresh fruit from your diet because you thought this might be helpful. Do not do this from theory: convince yourself first by several trials whether or not you can handle them.

Specific Food Intolerances and IBS

Many who suffer from IBS eliminate so many items from their diet, suspecting them of causing discomfort, that they end up eating very poor, unbalanced meals. Some few patients clearly have a limited tolerance for fiber and do better when salads or fruits are reduced or eliminated. This can be carried too far. For example, bananas are often well tolerated by some IBS sufferers, especially when ripe, but the haphazard elimination of one class of food after another is to be avoided. Only repeated trials should convince you that you really cannot tolerate salad or specific fruits. Most cooked or steamed vegetables can be eaten, but some people do better if the cabbage family of vegetables (cauliflower, kale, brussels sprouts, and cabbage) are eliminated. Beans obviously are known to be notorious for causing gas.

A few people have difficulty handling gluten, a protein that is present in wheat, rye, oats, and barley. Gluten can cause a severe diarrheal disorder in youngsters called *celiac disease* (Chapter 7), but some adults have a limited tolerance for gluten without suffering from celiac disease. They simply have a limited ability to handle wheat products. Such starches as wheat from bread, pasta, and cereals may fail to be completely absorbed in the small intestine in contrast to the starch derived from rice. As a result, some of the undigested carbohydrate, starches, enter the colon, where bacteria act on them and release gases that irritate the bowel. A trial of wheat withdrawal is sometimes in order.

The fear of eating specific foods because of suspected allergy or sensitivities can be carried too far and may lead to a deficient diet. In rare instances, where there is a documented family history of allergies or of allergic disorders such as hay fever, hives, or eczema, elimination diets may be tried. Indeed, many patients and not a few doctors are convinced that specific food intolerances play an important role in provoking some of the gastrointestinal symptoms of IBS. During the 1980s, the medical literature contained much on this disputed point, but much less emphasis is placed on food sensitivities in the therapy of IBS, at least by doctors nowadays.

Some rigorous studies, especially by our British colleagues, have thrown some light on the issue. In one careful study of 156 women with irritable bowel syndrome who were treated with dietary exclusion diets for three weeks, 48 percent showed symptomatic improvement. When they were challenged with individual foods, 73 of these 91 improved subjects were able to identify one or more food intolerances and 72 remained well on a modified diet during the follow-up period of about one year. Of the 98 patients who showed no symptomatic improvement after three weeks on the strict elimination diet, only 3 were symptomatically well in a follow-up of about eight months. There was no close correlation between the response and the types of symptoms reported.

In this study, the majority of subjects (50%) identified two to five foods that upset them. The foods most commonly incriminated were cereals, citrus fruits, potatoes, tea, coffee, alcohol, and additives, if any were known to be present. Other offenders included rich cheeses, onions, milk, wheat, chocolate, butter and yogurt, barley, oats, and corn. The authors of this study concluded that perhaps half of their patients improved by excluding certain foods from their diet, but the main problem was in the repeated failure of following these regimens. When my patients become desperate in their failure to find a suitable diet, sometimes, in my own desperation, I fall back on a "core" diet. For two or three weeks, I ask the patient to eat only one starch (rice), one protein (lamb or only chicken), one fruit (canned Bartlett pears), and to drink only bottled mineral water without carbonization before allowing the patient to add one new food at a time. Though tedious, this approach—called an *elimination diet*—may help individuals to pinpoint the offending food or drink, but obviously it is difficult to carry out in the midst of a busy workday. I've been most successful with patients who worked at home.

In this age of megavitamins, it is prudent to supplement your diet with an ordinary multivitamin tablet, one containing vitamins A, C, and E—megavitamin doses can be toxic and should be avoided. If you are avoiding milk and milk products, especially if you are a woman pre-or postpartum or postmenopause, supplementary calcium will be needed regularly.

Unfortunately, as you can see from this chapter's brevity, a dietary approach to the irritable bowel has not, in the majority of the cases, solved the patient's discomfort. Careful elimination diets have helped some, but we are far from having understood the basic physiological disturbance of the irritable bowel, which, as I have stated earlier, was in recent years considered to be a problem of altered motility or dysmotility of the intestinal tract. Now the emphasis has shifted to the increased sensitivity of the patient's nerves, transferring the origin of symptoms from the gut to the brain. A great deal of research is currently being devoted to this gut-brain connection, so we may expect help before too long.

9

❋ ❋ ❋

FOOD
INTOLERANCES
AND
FOOD ALLERGIES

In the previous chapter, we looked at the role that dietary intolerances may play in the cause and treatment of the irritable bowel syndrome, and it offers a convenient point of departure for a discussion of the whole area of food intolerances and food allergies. No area of gastrointestinal symptoms and gastrointestinal dietary advice is as difficult to present as the area of food intolerance and food allergies. All of us at some time or another have experienced some form of digestive discomfort after eating. "I am allergic to such-and-such" or "It must have been something I ate" are our frequent attempts to pinpoint these offenders.

How important are these food allergies? How many individuals suffer from them?

It is difficult to estimate the exact number of persons affected by food allergies. Estimates range all over the lot. *U.S.A. Today* recently stated that 60 percent of the population have a food allergy. The Asthma and Allergy Foundation states that about 1 percent of the entire American population is allergic to some food. The U.S. Department of Agriculture guesses the number ranges between 10 and 15 percent.

All too often we use the word *allergy* loosely. After a meal has made us uncomfortable, we take for granted that some food "doesn't agree with me." When we experience nausea, belching, burping, indigestion, dyspepsia, or heartburn in the upper abdomen or lower chest, followed by diarrhea and cramps in the lower abdomen, we declare, "I must be allergic to something I ate."

At times, we explain our gastrointestinal distress by claiming that we cannot tolerate this or that drink or food, and yet at other times we can eat and drink the same foodstuff without suffering any unpleasant reactions. We know that hay fever sufferers do not always sneeze when pollens are floating around because their threshold varies from time to time in response to the height of the pollen count.

Can we sort out these differences? In all this loose talk and thinking can we find some definite facts?

No one doubts that food allergies exist, but because controversy and possible quackery surround the whole subject, doctors approach it with great caution. The major problem is that it is difficult to prove that the symptoms blamed on food allergies are really caused by foods. Common symptoms include gastrointestinal complaints such as nausea, vomiting, abdominal cramps, and diarrhea; distant symptoms such as hives, swelling of the lips and throat, known as *angioneurotic edema*, and eczema; asthma and swelling of the nasal passages; and sometimes headache or migraine. With such a diverse list, you can see why your doctor might feel defeated even before beginning an investigation of possible causes.

Another reason why food allergies are difficult to identify is that the diagnostic tests are hard to interpret and unreliable. For example, "skin tests" in which extracts of the suspected foodstuffs are either pricked or scratched into the skin are widely used and equally widely suspected because they are unreliable. Recently, a great deal of energy and money has been spent on detailed chemical analyses of hair and fingernails in an effort to relate these findings to presumed nutritive deficiencies arising from disturbed diets. Although some understanding of the body's nutritional status, especially protein balance, can be gained from hair analysis, most of these expensive tests shed no real light on the nutritional problems being studied. Another group of tests that include radioallergosorbent tests (RASTs) and the measurement of immunoglobulins of the blood, especially immunoglobulin E (IgE), have a better scientific foundation but are expensive and often inconclusive. As a result, patients, physicians, and nutritionists resort to "elimination diets." Either specific foods (e.g., milk) or classes of food (e.g., wheat or dairy products) are forbidden or a few simple foods are allowed and new foodstuffs are gradually added to the diet. The elimination diet approach is widely used but difficult to follow given the daily demands placed on the actively employed individual.

Finally, food allergies are tricky to diagnose because the different kinds of reactions to food need to be separated and better defined. Recently, clinical researchers have made a start in this direction by attempting to improve and standardize the scientific bases of the classification of these reactions.

So it is not surprising that the general public and those who suspect they have food intolerances or allergies feel frustrated. Jane E. Brody, the noted and respected health columnist and science writer for the *New York Times*, in its magazine section of April 29, 1990, speaking for the public and for herself, pointed to growing controversies in this field and asked if doctors are paying enough attention to the problem.

Terms: Getting the Categories Straight

Food intolerance, the most widely used term, covers the whole gamut of adverse reactions to foods and includes two main groups of sufferers: those with *food idiosyncrasy* and those with *food allergy.*

Food idiosyncrasy refers to a specific reaction to a specific food substance, perhaps based on a specific defect in the body's enzyme system. *Phenylketonuria*, a disease in which the newborn infant cannot handle a specific amino acid and which is tested for routinely at birth, is such an example.

Food allergy refers to an adverse reaction to food that requires two criteria: (1) the participation of a component of the immune system (often quite difficult to prove), and (2) the recurrence of symptoms on two or more occasions when the suspected food is retested.

Yet it is often very difficult to decide whether an allergic reaction is present, even if you react badly every time you eat a specific substance. This gray area can include drugs as well as food. Aspirin sensitivity is a good example. The fact that some individuals react to aspirin with asthma or eczema suggests that an allergy is present, but the mechanics that cause the reaction have not been shown to be immunological—that is, involving the immune system.

Food intolerances that occur every time an individual eats or drinks a specific substance may be due to a direct *toxic chemical effect.* Rapid heartbeat after consuming tea, coffee, chocolate, or cocoa may result directly from the caffeine, theobromine, and methylxanthine in these substances.

With *lactose intolerance*, for example, individuals experience bloating, "gas," abdominal cramps, and even diarrhea after drinking milk or eating dairy products (e.g., cheese, ice cream, butter). Still other individuals, as they grow older, may develop these reactions to milk, although they did not experience them earlier in life. A considerable part of this intolerance to milk is due to the presence in milk of the sugar *lactose* (composed of one molecule of glucose and one molecule of galactose), which is split and digested by the enzyme *lactase*, present in the cells that line the intestinal tract. The lack or reduced amount of lactase allows some of the unsplit lactose to reach the colon, where the intestinal bacteria feed on it and produce gases and irritating acids. Lactose intolerance is now widely known by the general public. Those who need to drink milk can partially correct the lactase deficiency by adding a special enzyme preparation to the milk. Lactaid® is one such available remedy. The difficulties some people have with milk may also be related to other substances it contains, especially proteins. Milk contains at least twenty proteins and these can cause true allergic reactions.

Other substances such as wine may induce reactions because toxic materials are released when they are left to stand around after being opened. Foods that contain histamine, such as fermented cheeses and sausages, or that contain histamine-releasing tyramine, such as chocolate, cheeses, and canned fish, can also produce indications that mimic allergic reactions.

Another food intolerance most people have heard of is the *Chinese restaurant syndrome.* Characterized by gastric distress, warmth, flushing, headaches, and dizziness, this reaction is presumed to result from monosodium glutamate (MSG) contained in Chinese dishes. Symptoms often appear within thirty minutes after eating.

The additive and preservative *sulfite* can also cause reactions. Because of this sensitivity, wines and other products that contain sulfites must be clearly labeled. The reaction to sulfites includes headache, dizziness, and stomach distress.

As you can imagine, the list of foods suspected of causing allergic symptoms is long. In one study of 100 patients, the following foods were tested for sensitivity; the number of individuals claiming sensitivity to the food is given in parentheses: milk (46), eggs (40), nuts/peanuts (22), fish/shellfish (22), wheat-flour (9), tea and coffee (8), chocolate (8), artificial colors (7), pork/bacon (7), and chicken, tomatoes, soft fruit, and cheese (6 each).

In a more recent report, another group of about 200 individuals who could identify a specific food intolerance were tested; the following percentage of individuals complained of these foodstuffs: cheese, 35 percent; onions, 35; milk, 34; wheat, 30; chocolate, 30; butter, 25; yogurt, 25; coffee, 24; eggs, 23; nuts, 17; citrus fruits, 18; tea, 18; rye, 18; potatoes, 15; barley, 13; oats, 12; corn, 11; alcohol, 7; fruit, 8; yeast, 6; vegetables, 6; red meat, 4; salads, 2; spicy foods, 2; additives and saccharin, 2; bran, 1; and fat, 1 percent.

Products that contain mold spores may also be a problem, and these would include highly aged cheese, wine, yogurt, and yeast.

A True Allergic Reaction

Experiencing symptoms such as swelling of the lips or tongue, a runny nose, hives, asthma, or eczema, within minutes of eating a certain food, is clear evidence of an allergic reaction.

If your symptoms begin more than an hour after eating the suspected food, it is more difficult to prove that they are caused by an allergy. The first thing to do is to be certain that these symptoms recur every time you eat the suspected substance. In addition to the symptoms mentioned above, those that may appear more than an hour after a particular food is consumed include such gastrointestinal effects as vomiting, diarrhea, abdominal pain, bloating, and constipation. In rare cases, intestinal bleeding may be part of an allergic reaction. To rule out an intestinal disorder that can cause the same symptoms, your doctor should first take a careful history, give you a complete physical examination, and request the appropriate laboratory tests of gastrointestinal structures.

Wheat Intolerance

Wheat or substances that contain the wheat protein called gluten, such as wheat-containing flour, bread, cakes, stuffings, pasta, and so on, appear frequently on the list of substances people cannot tolerate. Gluten is present also in rye, oats, and barley.

One disease, *sprue*, or *gluten enteropathy*, to use its technical label, is a form of intestinal malabsorption that is clearly due to the inability of the individual's intestinal lining cells to handle gluten (Chapter 7). This leads to malabsorption, weight loss, loss of fat in the stools, and often diarrhea and bloating. A chronic skin condition, *dermatitis herpetiformis*, known as *Duhring's disease*, may also be associated with sprue or sprue-like changes in the small intestine. The striking point here is that removal of gluten from the diet leads to prompt restoration of health and the disappearance of symptoms. The diagnosis rests not only on the good effect of withdrawing gluten from the diet, but on the fact that biopsies of the small intestinal lining reveal marked abnormalities that return to normal as the individual's health improves. In a few cases, people with sprue need to remove lactose from their diets as well. Very rarely, even removal of these two major offenders is not enough, and other substances such as chicken and eggs must be eliminated from the diet as well.

We still don't know whether the sensitivity to gluten in sprue is purely an allergic (immunologically mediated) reaction or is also in part a toxic chemical reaction. Before the discovery in the 1960s of wheat's role in sprue, this disorder was treated with cortisone that suppressed a presumed immunological inflammation in the intestinal wall. Unlike sprue, mild wheat intolerance does not inflame the cell lining of the intestine, but it does cause intestinal symptoms such as bloating, gas, distention, and even diarrhea. There is no laboratory test to prove this condition, only the reactions of the individual to repeated attempts to eat wheat or wheat-containing foodstuffs.

Although almost everything we eat that is digested by the intestinal secretions is completely absorbed by the body, some starch is not broken down by the appropriate enzymes, escapes absorption in the small bowel, and reaches the colon. The amount varies from individual to individual and depends on the kind of starch. For example, the carbohydrate of rice flour is absorbed completely, whereas some of the carbohydrate of all-purpose white wheat flour is not. This malabsorption in some individuals can be corrected by withdrawing gluten from the diet.

This curious phenomenon is thought to be caused by an interaction between starch and wheat protein, which interferes with the former's complete absorption and thus produces unpleasant gut sensations. Until we understand this problem better, however, it is important not to fall victim to the many untested remedies that have been proposed, such as eating certain substances only with certain other substances; you risk developing a lopsided diet.

Can Complex Carbohydrates Cause Discomfort?

Some progress has been made with specific food allergies. I have already discussed some of the defects in digesting particular carbohydrates in the previous chapter on irritable bowel syndrome. These complex carbohydrates or sugars include sorbitol and fructose. Sorbitol is found in some fruit juices, especially apple juice, and pediatricians have recently pointed out that some infants have diarrhea from sorbitol-containing fruit juices. Some candies prepared for overweight individuals to reduce their caloric intake also contain considerable amounts of sorbitol and cause diarrhea. No digestive enzymes are available that can improve your indigestion if these complex sugars are the cause. They must be eliminated from the diet.

If your intestine does not absorb these complex carbohydrates, you will experience the effects of the fermentation of these starches in the colon. When these sugars escape absorption in the small bowel, excessive gas will build up and cause individuals considerable discomfort. We can appreciate the relative importance of this introduced starch to the colon if we realize that the amount of malabsorbed fermentable material from a 100-gram diet may exceed 20 grams from baked beans, 7 to 10 grams from wheat, oats, potatoes, and corn, and very little from rice—less than 1 gram. Whole oats and whole wheat result in two times the normal fermentable material in the colon. So it is clear that some individuals may be uncomfortable from complex starches that fail to be absorbed in the small bowel. Rice in this situation is handled better than oats, whole wheat, potatoes, corn, or baked beans. This is not, however, an all-or-none phenomenon. These guidelines vary from individual to individual and will vary with the amount of these substances that is eaten. You must try to reduce your starch intake if this is your trouble. Some individuals can be cured by eliminating gluten, wheat, rye, oats, and barley to varying degrees.

Newly Understood Food Allergies

Shellfish

While information about a specific food intolerance or bowel syndrome is hard won, researchers in the United States and India have successfully identified the protein component that causes the well-known allergy to shrimp. The protein tropomyosin is found in the muscle of these creatures, and it attaches to two areas of the antibody E, which is the major blood marker for allergic reactions. It is hoped that this discovery of one of the few allergenic foods for which an allergen has been discovered and purified may lead to methods of desensitizing individuals so they may someday enjoy shrimp. Of the individuals who have documented food allergies to peanuts, shellfish, tree nuts, eggs, and other seafoods, about one-quarter of these people are allergic to shellfish and develop a reaction ranging from itching of the mouth to more serious problems—trouble breathing and swallowing, as well as abdominal pain and diarrhea. A person allergic to shrimp is also likely to react adversely to lobster, crab, and other crustaceans that have similar tropomyosins as the one identified in shrimp. But people may vary intensely in their allergies to shellfish. Dr. Dean Metcalfe of The National Institute of Allergy and Infectious Diseases has seen one patient who suffered a reaction on being in a room where shrimp was being boiled, and another whose lips would swell if she kissed her boyfriend after he ate shrimp. Dr. Metcalfe recommends that these very allergic people should carry syringes of epinephrine (adrenalin) to use in case they suffer severe reactions, especially since they may be exposed to these allergenic substances unknowingly.

Peanuts

It may be helpful to devote some space to the problem of individuals with a serious peanut allergy. While these persons are careful to avoid a peanut butter sandwich, they have gotten ill from inadvertent exposure to peanuts in egg rolls or graham cracker pie crusts. One does not outgrow an allergy to peanuts and will suffer an extremely severe reaction call *anaphylaxis*, essentially a vascular collapse and difficulty in breathing, from the effect of the peanut protein on the immune system. Ginger snaps and protein potato chips can set off such a reaction. Even a particle of a peanut can create real trouble.

An accidental exposure with its life-threatening risk should be treated. A self-injection kit containing epinephrine (adrenalin) is available by prescription under such names as EpiPen® or ANA Kit®. Susceptible individuals who are aware of this possibility should carry one of these kits around with them and use it in the case of a suspected exposure.

The Food Allergy Network, founded by Anne Mumnoz-Furing, tries to keep track of the products that contain peanut protein in any form. The network is located at 10400 Eaton Place, Suite 107, Fairfax, Virginia 22030, telephone: (703) 691-3179.

10

❋ ❋ ❋

DIARRHEA AND
CONSTIPATION

Definitions

My definitions are quite simple. By *diarrhea* I mean bowel movements that occur too often and that are too loose. By *constipation* I mean difficulty in moving one's bowels (although some people think they are constipated if their bowel movements are dry and hard; these are not necessarily signs of constipation). Again, difficulty in moving one's bowels is the important symptom.

To put the definitions of diarrhea and constipation in proper perspective, the number of bowel movements that normal people in good health can pass varies tremendously, ranging from two to three per day to two to three per week. However, perfectly normal individuals may have many fewer or many more bowel movements than these average numbers. One should look for deviations from one's ordinary routines both in number and consistency of the stool.

Diarrhea

Acute Diarrhea ("Intestinal Virus")

From time to time, we all suffer episodes of gastrointestinal upset in which we are nauseated, vomit, and have diarrhea. We
can't recall a specific meal or food that may have caused the
episode. Other members of our family may have similar discomfort, but we are not part of an epidemic "going around," nor are
we one of a group that went to the same banquet or picnic. The
upset is usually mild, but occasionally can be more severe.
Many times we have some fever accompanying our discomfort,
lots of loose stools, sometimes mucus, but not blood. We are
quite uncomfortable, and yet the whole episode is usually over
in three to four days. We may not even call our doctor. We have
had these bouts before; we are prepared to wait this one out.
When asked what was wrong with us, we pass it off as an "intestinal virus." This kind of illness is the second most common
clinical sickness in our society. Babies as well as adults have it,
and travelers of industrialized countries visiting developing
countries are especially susceptible. This group of diarrhea sufferers deserves special attention, but stay-at-homes get it also.

What causes common episodes of gastrointestinal upset? Infectious agents—viruses, bacteria, or parasites—are responsible
for most acute episodes of gastroenteritis and are spread mainly
by food or water contaminated by persons, animals, or the environment that contains the culprit; these agents can also be
transmitted by person-to-person contact.

The viruses that attack infants and babies are mainly of the
rota virus group or the Norwalk agent. In adults, the bacteria
includes specific types of *E. coli*, which produces a toxin, but
the majority of bacteria are of the salmonella, Shigella, *Yersinia
enterocolitica*, and campylobacter families. In the case of the
last named, a sick household pet, such as a puppy, is frequently
the source of the infection.

What about treatment for acute episodes? For most individuals with acute milder diarrhea, the episodes are self-limited and one gets over the virus without medication. In the more severe cases, replacement of the fluid and electrolyte loss in the gut is essential—by mouth, if you can take fluids; intravenously, if you cannot. For symptomatic relief, three groups of medicines are frequently prescribed: (1) subsalicylates in the United States in the form of Pepto-Bismol®, which cuts down the secretions of the intestine but turns the stool black; (2) loperamide (Imodium®) or diphenoxylate (Lomotil®), which slows down the movement of the intestine and its secretion but may worsen the disease by retarding the evacuation of the organisms responsible; and finally, (3) nonabsorbable earth mixtures of kaolin and pectin (in the U.S. Kaopectate®). This last group of medications is harmless and makes the stools more bulky, but probably does little else.

Of the bacterial causes, most cases of salmonella are not treated with antibiotics, unless your bloodstream has been invaded by parasites. Then ampicillin or Cipro® is the drug of choice. For others (*E. coli*, Shigella, or campylobacter), antibiotics of the sulfa group, especially the mixture of trimethoprim and sulfamethoxozol (Bactrim®, Septra®), or erythromycin are prescribed.

The viral forms are rarely demonstrated with laboratory tests. We have no specific medicines, and except in the case of dehydrated infants, these patients need no hospitalization or intravenous fluids. The viral infections usually subside in a few days.

What Do I Eat during an Acute Episode of Diarrhea? For a mild case of diarrhea, I advise a cooked diet, nothing raw, with the elimination even of steamed vegetables. For the more severe forms, clear liquids seem most helpful: clear broth, tea, jello, bottled noncarbonated water, and liquid drinks such as Gaterade. As the diarrhea subsides, you may start to add other soft foods: cooked cereal, baked or mashed potato, going on to baked or boiled chicken, fish, soft boiled eggs, or canned fruit. Milk

Table 9. Common Food-Borne Illnesses

Carrier	Organism
Beef	*E. coli* Salmonella *Staphylococcus aureus*
Ham/pork	Salmonella
Poultry	Salmonella *Campylobacter jejuni* *Staphylococcus aureus*
Eggs	Salmonella *Staphylococcus aureus*
Cheese	*E. coli* Salmonella
Fish/shellfish	*Clostridium botulinum* *Vibrio cholerae* Salmonella
Fried rice	*Bacillus cereus*

should be resumed only after several days, along with other dairy products, and steamed vegetables (avoiding the cabbage family). Raw fruit and salad should be the last foods resumed.

What about Food Poisoning? We only think about an episode of food poisoning when more than one individual experiences the same illness shortly after partaking of the same food. These episodes are mostly caused by some of the bacteria already mentioned in this section and by toxins produced by bacterial organisms. In many instances, a specific agent is not identified for technical reasons or because the suspected foods are no longer available for testing. One may suspect that a particular organism has caused the outbreak because it is associated with a common food prone to carry the organism. A list of these foods is provided in Table 9 titled "Common Food-Borne Illnesses." Dietary treatment is the same as that outlined for an acute episode of diarrhea.

Traveler's Diarrhea

Nowadays millions of people traveling throughout the world run the risk of developing *traveler's diarrhea* (TD), which usually translates into twice the number of stools daily as well as loose stools. Most of us have experienced this in one or more forms. Usually the attack manifests itself while we are abroad or soon after we get home. We may experience abdominal cramps, nausea, bloating, the need to empty our bowels in a hurry, a generally sick feeling, and sometimes a fever. On rare occasions, the diarrhea may become violent and may be accompanied by rectal bleeding. Most people get over traveler's diarrhea rapidly by themselves without any particular prescriptions.

How Can We Avoid Getting Traveler's Diarrhea? There are no vaccines at present for the organisms that cause TD. Thus caution and meticulous attention to where and what you eat and drink are the best preventive measures. The use of Lomotil® (diphenoxylate) or Imodium® (loperamide) does not prevent TD, though most traveler's carry and use them. Bismuth subsalicylate, however, the active ingredient of Pepto-Bismol® taken in liquid form, two ounces four times a day, has prevented some travelers from developing TD, but taking large doses of bismuth subsalicylate for a two- to three-week trip not only means carrying a huge supply but may be risky. Most doctors advise against this, and so do I.

A few antibiotics, such as doxycycline (Vibromycin®), and the mixed sulfas (Bactrim® and Septra®) taken as precautionary measures can often reduce the chance of developing TD. But there are side effects including colitis associated with antibiotics that often lead me to advise against their preventive use. The common side effects include sun rashes, sensitivity to sunlight, bowel disorders, and fungal infections of the vagina. The risks are just too great to hand out these drugs to all travelers who might develop TD.

Table 10. Areas of Risk for Traveler's Diarrhea

Low-Risk Area	Moderate or Unknown Risk Area	High-Risk Area
Australia	Albania	Afghanistan
Austria	Argentina	Africa (all
Belgium	Bulgaria	countries except
Canada	Caribbean Islands	South Africa)
Denmark	(other than Haiti and	Bangladesh
Finland	Dominican Republic)	Cambodia
France	Chile	Central America
Germany	China	(all countries)
Ireland	Cuba	Dominican Republic
Isle of Man	Cyprus	Haiti
Japan	Czechoslovakia	India
Liechtenstein	Greece	Indonesia
Luxembourg	Greenland	Iran
Monaco	Hong Kong	Iraq
Netherlands	Hungary	Korea
New Zealand	Iceland	Laos
Norway	Israel	Mexico
South Africa	Italy	Myanmar (Burma)
Sweden	Jordan	Nepal
Switzerland	Pacific Islands	New Guinea
United Kingdom	Poland	Pakistan
United States	Portugal	Philippines
	Romania	Saudi Arabia
	Russia	South America (all
	Spain	countries)
	Taiwan	Sri Lanka
	Tasmania	Syria
	Yugoslavia	Thailand
		Turkey
		Vietnam

Source: Herbert L. DuPont, M.D. and Margaret W. DuPont, M.A., *Travel with Health*, New York, Appleton Century-Crofts, 1981.

What Treatment Works for Traveler's Diarrhea? Although for most travelers TD is a nuisance and not a serious illness, we all want relief from cramps and diarrhea. A large number of popular methods have been used over the years to absorb the toxic agents of TD—activated charcoal, for example—but they don't work. Kaopectate® gives the stool a firmer consistency but otherwise does not help a lot. Drugs that combat diarrhea work by slowing down the bowel and have been used for a long time. The newest of these synthetic agents—Lomotil® and Imodium®—give temporary symptomatic comfort but should not be continued if the symptoms persist for more than a few days. Travelers should remember that Pepto-Bismol® turns the stool black and that the changing color is not due to blood in the stool. Aspirin should be avoided while taking Pepto-Bismol®, since both in combination may irritate the stomach.

It is also important to replace the fluid lost from the intestines with TD and to avoid getting dehydrated. Milk and dairy products should be avoided. If you are mildly dehydrated, you should drink potable fruit juices, caffeine-free soda drinks, consomme, and safe water. Salty crackers can be used to nibble on. More dehydrated individuals may find solutions such as Gatorade, Lucozade, or mineral water with added sugar useful. In the severer forms that resemble cholera, you may need some mixture of electrolytes in water that can be given by mouth or even intravenously. You will need to consult a physician to obtain these.

If you are sicker than most travelers with symptoms involving fever, severe pain, or even bloody stools, antibiotics can help shorten the illness. The sulfa drug trimethoprim or the combination sulfas (Bactrim®, Septra®) for no more than three to five days are useful. Recently, a single dose of Cipro® has been found helpful for these sufferers.

In all these situations, care must be taken if the individual is a child or a pregnant woman. Kaolin and pectin (Kaopectate®) are harmless, but try to get by without the other medications if you are pregnant. Tetracycline can stain the teeth of children under 12, and the sulfa combinations may cause a skin rash and sensitivity to sunlight in all ages.

Parasites

Even in the United States, and even if the patient is not very sick, it is important to have the stool examined for parasites if a person is suffering from mild but chronic diarrhea. *Entamoeba histolytica* and *Giardia lamblia* can be difficult to find so the search must be very diligent. One does not have to go to the tropics to pick up the organism. It is as easy to get it in New York City as on a tropical isle. Giardiasis is notorious in certain parts of the world and epidemics have originated in Aspen, Colorado; Zurich, Switzerland; and St. Petersburg. The secret to finding parasites lies in fresh stools, preferably passed directly in the lab or brought directly from home and examined before they dry out. The testing may require several examinations or at least up to three to exclude infection with the amoeba, although a blood test may help in suggesting exposure to a parasite. Smears of the stool taken directly through a sigmoidoscope may reveal the organism if stained appropriately. *Giardia lamblia* will also cause some nausea along with diarrhea and is quite elusive because it lives in the upper intestine and may not be seen in every stool specimen. In suspected cases, it may be necessary to obtain juice from your duodenum by passing a tube through the mouth to that area. On rare occasions, both of these organisms may be found embedded in the tissues of the duodenum and colon, and biopsies are done in a specific search for them. Tedious as the search for these parasites may be for patient and doctor, it is clearly worth the effort in eliminating these chronic "boarders" in the intestine. The drug metronidazole (Flagyl®) will usually cure the condition.

Secretory Diarrhea

Some forms of diarrhea have nothing to do with eating but are
due to fluids secreted by the intestine; these are called *secretory
diarrheas.* These may be caused by a small hidden tumor spe-
cifically in the pancreas which releases chemical messengers
that stimulate the bowel to pour out fluid. Though secretory
diarrheas are quite rare, and those caused by tumors are among
the rarest, it is important to remember that certain medications
can mimic these symptoms. The drugs that most commonly
cause secretory diarrhea and often the hardest to detect are laxatives and "water pills" (diuretics). These are harder to detect
because individuals take them secretly, usually in a desperate
attempt to lose weight.

Food Intolerance as a Cause of Diarrhea

But what about the "harmless" things we eat? *Intolerance* to
lactose, the sugar in milk, discussed in Chapter 8 on "Irritable Bowel Syndrome," certainly can give some individuals
frequent and loose stools. Beyond this, a whole list of foods
are blamed by different people as the cause of their diarrhea.
There certainly is biochemical individuality, just as there are
individual personalities. One must be careful about eliminating one food after another because of "suspected" food intolerance and food allergies. From a statistical point of view,
milk, egg, and wheat are the most likely offenders. Some
people have a limited ability to digest and absorb starch, and
there are curious interactions between starches and wheat.
You want to avoid a lopsided diet by eliminating one food
after another without some proof that these foods really are
causing you chronic diarrhea. Here the guidance of a doctor
is really important.

Antibiotic-Associated Diarrhea

Few of us have reached adulthood without having endured a bout of cramps and diarrhea after receiving an antibiotic. There is practically speaking no antibiotic that has not been associated with diarrhea following its use by mouth or by vein. Most episodes are shortlived, moderate in their severity, and respond quite favorably and promptly when the antibiotic is stopped. Occasionally, however, the effect of the antibiotic is more severe and persists even after the drug has been discontinued.

In recent years it has been learned that antibiotics interfere with the ecology of the gut; they suppress some natural inhabitants and favor the growth of other bacteria which lie dormant in the colon. This is especially true of the *Claustra* genus. When one type of this organism becomes rampant and secretes two toxins, *C. difficile* toxins A, B, it directly injures the intestinal lining, forming false membranes (pseudomembranous colitis) and stimulating the bowel to secrete large amounts of fluid containing important salts of the blood (sodium and potassium).

To combat *C. difficile* toxins, the organism must be eliminated from the bowel by other antagonistic antibiotics, such as vancomycin or metronidazole (Flagyl®), or neutralized by the resin cholestyramine that binds the toxins. The bacteria of this group are hardy individuals and stubborn to eradicate.

During treatment, eating should follow the course I have outlined for the severe form of diarrhea: clear fluids at first, followed by all liquids, including thin cooked cereal, and then soft foods without any fiber.

Constipation

The simplest definition of constipation is difficulty in moving one's bowels. More precisely, it is needing to strain to have a bowel movement more than 25 percent of the time. What is "normal" varies tremendously. Although normal individuals move their bowels between three times a day and three times a week, many others move their bowels more or less frequently, some as seldom as every three to five or even nine days, and some more often than three times a day.

We all may have experienced short periods of constipation whatever definition we use. Accustomed to our own routine, we may have temporary difficulty on a trip if we don't have access to our own bathroom. But when this difficulty persists, we become uncomfortable and worry about its meaning, in part because doctors have alerted everyone to pay attention to any change in bowel habits in an effort to diagnose cancer of the colon at an earlier and more treatable stage. The main point to remember is that change alone is not important; we all may have a temporary change in bowel habits. What is important is *persistent* change.

If you do experience persistent constipation, stop to consider whether you are taking any new medicines before you contact your doctor. A great many drugs, especially those for the control of high blood pressure, can effect the motility of the colon. Other drugs that cause constipation include painkillers containing codeine, morphine, or opium in any form, antacid compounds, and many psychotropic drugs such as the mood elevators and those used to treat parkinsonism. Iron by itself as a pill or in vitamin mixtures can cause the stool to become dark, almost black, induce cramps, and constipate some individuals. Medications that cause constipation are easily remedied; with the consent of your doctor, you can use a substitute drug without this annoying but harmless side effect.

Another thing to consider is whether you have for some reason cut down the amount of fiber you are eating by reducing your intake of fruits, salads, fresh vegetables, and cereal carbohydrates.

What Is the Usual Cause of Constipation, and How Is It Treated?

The most common cause of constipation in the Western world is inadequate fiber and roughage in the diet. It has been clearly demonstrated that in other parts of the world, Africa especially, with a native population that lives on a diet high in unrefined carbohydrates, constipation, the irritable bowel, even diverticular disease and cancer of the colon are much less frequently seen than in the developed countries of the West. As a result, current treatment of constipation calls for a marked increase in dietary fiber in the form of certain vegetables, raw fruits, nuts, flour, and especially cereals. Tremendous emphasis has been given to taking bran and certain plant seeds, namely psyllium seeds, which are the active part of Metamucil® and related products.

What Is Dietary Fiber?

Even experts have trouble defining this term. It includes all the complex plant carbohydrates that cannot be digested in the intestine by our digestive enzymes; this means all those substances that enter the colon undigested. In the normal small intestine, almost all food substances and most lipids and vitamins are completely absorbed. But some water and its components (salts of sodium and potassium, and vitamins) and the undigested residues of plant foods enter the colon. A small part of some starches—potato, wheat, rice, etc.—escape small bowel digestion as well.

Once fiber enters the colon, the local bacteria add bulk to the stool and increase its water and gas content by fermentation. Just how fiber does this is far from agreed upon. Formerly it was thought that the increase in the bulk of stool was due solely to the water-holding action of intact fiber, but this explanation is not accepted nowadays. It may be due to the stool's increased bacterial contents, since these intestinal organisms can and do live on fibrous material (half of the normal stool is made up of bacteria). Fiber also hastens the transit time from the colon and lowers pressure in the lower colon, and perhaps this allows the contents to pass through more easily and faster.

Treatment with High-Fiber Diets

I highly recommend a high-fiber diet to those who are constipated and urge them to eat the raw fruits and vegetables listed in Table 3. In addition to fiber content, some foods such as prunes and figs contain naturally occurring substances that simulate intestinal evacuation. An old-fashioned plant, senna, was used by our grandmothers and our great-grandmothers in the form of a tea (more recently, senna has been marketed in a standardized form, commercially known as Senokot®). The switch to a high-fiber diet is often hard for some people to adapt to, and their intestine may need time to adjust to the new diet as well, but the bowels will be stimulated to empty themselves more easily.

Working on the High-Fiber Diet

The first thing to do before starting the high-fiber diet is to do an inventory of what fiber you are actually eating. You may be like many people. Because they eat some salad and fruit, they believe they are on a high-fiber diet. You will need to keep track of everything you eat over a three-day period, listing the food and a rough estimate of the amount. (I refer you to Table 3.) You can make a calculation of the actual amount of fiber in your daily customary diet. For most individuals who really need lots of fiber, it is quite startling to find out that the foods they do eat contain very little fiber. Most of the experts in this field agree we should all aim for between 25 and 35 grams of fiber daily, and most of us don't consume anywhere near that amount.

You can see from Table 3 that meats, poultry, eggs, and dairy products contain absolutely no fiber, and many fruits have very little (strawberries and blackberries, curiously enough, have lots). Green vegetables vary tremendously from very little in a cup of raw spinach to 3.5 grams in a half-cup of broccoli. Raisins and crackers do not contain very much fiber content. But cereals, especially the brans, have the highest amount.

Once you embark on a high-fiber diet, it will become clear to you that you are going to have to work at it to achieve the desired amount in your daily intake. It is not easy. Eating in restaurants and fast-food places until recently also presented obstacles, but now that the value of the high-fiber diet in reducing a whole host of disorders has become better known in our society, salad bars and vegetable platters have been multiplying. It still will not be easy until your high-fiber intake becomes an automatic habit.

In addition to the plant seed supplements in your diet, another way of getting enough fiber into your daily food intake is to eat fiber cookies. Fiber-Med® and Fiber-Rich® are two of the commercially available forms sold in drugstores and supermarkets. These contain about 5 grams of fiber in each cracker and are rather palatable. My simple rule is to add one new substance at each meal and to slow down if you get unpleasant symptoms from your intestines—rumbling, gas, and any discomfort. Don't give up. Stay with it. Your bowels will adjust.

More about Bran

Bran in its natural raw-milled form, often called *Miller's bran*, is a very good source of fiber, and 1 ounce can give you quite a lot. A simple way to take it is to add it to your usual cereal, shake it onto cottage cheese, or mix it in with your yogurt. Individuals vary and some cannot tolerate much or even small amounts of bran. If after a real try you find you are one of these people, then give up trying bran. The other forms of fiber will do just as well. For those of us who cannot tolerate bran, the psyllium seed preparations are excellent substitutes. There are a number of these preparations easily available. Perhaps the best known is Metamucil®, which comes either in bulk pack-ages or in small individual packets. These preparations are not too unpalatable. You can drink them with water or in fruit juices. The best time to take them is before going to bed, and as with all medications, the dose must be adjusted to each indi-vidual.

What about Lubricants?

Lubricants, of which mineral oil is generally the best known, are not absorbed in the intestine and thus supply oil to the in-testinal tract where they can lubricate the hard stool in the colon in the chronically constipated person. Nowadays lubricants are frowned on because they are habit forming, interfere with the absorption of certain vitamins (those that dissolve in fat), and may be inhaled into the lungs, especially in youngsters.

A more accepted form of lubricant is sodium dioctyl sulfate which is sold by prescription as Colase®. It can also be bought over the counter as Surfak®. One does not want to become de-pendent on these substances, although they are harmless.

For those individuals who have lost the sensations that re-mind us to defecate or whose awareness of these sensations has been blunted by years of constipation or the use of laxatives, sometimes simple nonmedicated suppositories that restore rec-tal sensation may do the trick. The suppositories that depend on irritating chemicals—for instance, Dulcolax®—should be avoided, except on rare isolated occasions. (They are of the type used in preparing the colon for X-ray examination.) Sometimes the substance lactulose, a nonabsorbable carbohydrate that stimulates water to enter the intestine, may help to lubricate the stool and is nonirritating.

What about Enemas?

Although it is not a good idea to become dependent on artificial stimulation to start off a bowel movement, of all the local stimulants the simple tap-water enema, placed in the rectum using warm tap-water by means of a baby bulb syringe, is certainly the most harmless. This kind of enema mimics the natural distention of the rectum by stool and sets off the reflex by which the rectum empties itself as the "trap door" muscles or sphincters open themselves.

Fluid Intake

Many people do not understand how liquids in the diet may affect bowel movements. In a healthy person, the body's requirements for fluid are closely regulated by thirst. If you satisfy your thirst and your kidneys are normal, you will take in enough water and put out enough urine. The fluid content of your diet cannot wash out your colon because the small bowel absorbs most of the liquids we drink, and only a small amount enters the colon. Ordinarily, the small intestine absorbs water so efficiently that even a slight disturbance caused by illness can overwhelm the colon's ability to handle the fluid load. Attempts to liquify hard stools by increased fluid intake rarely work, unless your "normal" intake of fluids in all forms (milk, tea, coffee, soups, water, soft drinks, etc.) has been grossly deficient.

More about Fiber's Benefits

Since there is so much interest in fiber nowadays (and I predict we will be even more concerned with fiber in the future), I want to add a little more information for those who are interested. Many terms are used for this class of plant materials that are not digested by the secretions of the human intestinal tract: *unavailable carbohydrates, nonnutritive fiber, nonedible fiber. Dietary fiber* remains, in my opinion, the most useful label.

The chemical structure of these fibrous materials does not concern us here. Known as celluloses, hemicelluloses, pectin, or lignins—all are present in the tissues of vegetables, fruits, apple peels, potato skins, and cereals. These dietary fibers have a great water-holding capacity. A hundred grams of turnip fiber will hold 1 ounce of water, but the same amount of bran fiber will hold up to 15 ounces of water. These fibers affect the rate at which materials pass through the intestinal tract, increase the bulk of our stools, and bind bile and the products of fat digestion. We are just beginning to learn what they do within the whole range of intestinal, digestive, and absorptive functions.

Fiber in our diet can interfere with the enzymes that digest fat by "tying" them up, so to speak, thus reducing the amount of fat that can be absorbed. This results in a loss of fat and cholesterol in the stool and a lowering of these amounts in the blood. This is clearly the case with oat bran, but corn bran and beans probably act in a different way in reducing blood cholesterol. So you see why in the current attempts to reduce heart attacks the emphasis on fiber is so important. Before fats can be digested and absorbed, these fibers bind parts of the bile needed to dissolve fats. Thus fiber is not only good for our bowel but good for our heart.

Although we cannot digest the complex carbohydrates of dietary fiber, the bacteria of the colon can. Some of this digestion may be useful by releasing the constituents of mucus, which could replenish the protective jellylike coating of the colon. On the other hand, bacteria can release gases in the colon that result from the process of fermentation and can create discomfort. You can appreciate why the effects of dietary fiber on the action of intestinal bacteria are being studied so intensively at present, especially their role in preventing tumors of the colon. Fiber prevents bacteria from altering the bile salts that do reach the colon. These salts are thought to play a part in triggering the cancerous process in the colon.

Not only the fats of our blood, but our blood sugar as well, can be lowered by the dietary fiber we eat. Carbohydrates taken in fiber meals produce a lower blood-sugar level, lower than those without fiber. In diabetics, for instance, fiber lowers the requirements for insulin. This seems to be due to the effect of fiber on the stomach and intestines. At both sites, fiber slows the absorption of sugar. Interestingly enough, a fiber meal at breakfast has a carryover effect, lowering sugars taken at lunchtime as well. Even more interesting, kidney beans, red lentils, and soybeans (the group known as *legumes*) are better for us than bread, rice, or potatoe in lowering blood sugar levels.

11

✳ ✳ ✳

DIVERTICULA, DIVERTICULOSIS, AND DIVERTICULITIS

In this chapter, I want to address the role of diet in preventing and treating those curious little pouches that can occur along the gastrointestinal tract, mostly in the colon, that are at times painful, and that sometimes can cause serious complications. I'll have a word to say as well about those pouches that cluster in the small intestine, particularly the jejunum.

These little pouches, called *diverticula* (singular diverticulum), are composed of two outer layers of smooth muscle that line the entire small and large bowel. When pressure rises in the bowel as the muscles contract to move their contents along, these thin-walled sacs balloon through the outer wall. The place where these diverticula appear is not a matter of chance. They form in areas of potential weakness, where the blood vessels, which supply the nutrient and oxygen requirements to the colon, enter the bowel and pierce its wall. These are the points of least resistance and the sacs bulge outward here.

Who Gets Diverticulosis?

Most are adults in their forties and fifties, although they do occur in younger and older individuals. There may be as many as 10 to 15 percent of individuals in Western nations studied by X-ray who have these pouches. Once these develop, they do not seem to multiply or disappear, and seem to retain their basic distribution. Because these pockets need room to expand outside the muscle walls of the colon, they can only occur in that part of the bowel that lies within the peritoneal cavity of the abdomen.

What Part of the Colon Suffers Most?

The diverticula are most frequent in the sigmoid colon, least frequent in the cecum, and appear scattered across the transverse colon. This does not mean that they cannot occur in the cecum, because they do on occasion, but only with considerable rarity.

In order for potential diverticula to become active ones, the wall of the sigmoid colon must react to increased pressure, and like any other muscle of the body, the colonic muscle reacts by getting thicker, which results in a thickened colonic wall with a few diverticula.

You must remember that the colon is essentially a cylindrical tank of varying width, the cecal area being the widest and the sigmoid area being the narrowest. The transverse colon is of intermediate diameter.

You may remember from your high school physics that the pressure in the wall of a cylinder varies inversely with its diameter: the wider the diameter, the lower the pressure; the narrower the diameter of the cylinder, the higher the pressure. This explains why the diverticula tend to accumulate more in the sigmoid area, a narrow passage. Theoretically, therefore, as the narrow segments of the colon have their diameter widened, the pressure in the wall of the segment is lowered and the chances of developing diverticula are lessened. On the other hand, if the pressure of the diameter of the narrow segments is unchanged, then the possibility of developing diverticula increases. The wide diameter of the cecum explains why this area is spared the most.

What Led to the Recognition that Diet Is an Important Factor in This Condition?

This insight was mainly the work and clever thinking of one individual, Dr. D. P. Burkett, an English physician working in Africa. He realized that diverticulosis varies in different parts of the world—and is rare in parts of the undeveloped and emerging nations, such as certain areas in Africa. Burkett hypothesized that this was probably related to the nature of their diet and its influence on sigmoid diameter, and not related merely to the extent of the sigmoid incidence of pouches. The striking feature of their diet was its very high-fiber content.

How Does Fiber Affect These Pouches?

As the diameter of the narrowed segment of the colon is widened by the bulk of the diet, the pressure in the wall automatically falls, decreasing the risk of developing diverticula. It is essentially the bulk of the colonic content and its fiber that influence the colon in this condition.

Remember that the diverticula of the colon develop in areas of potential weakness, where blood vessels enter the wall. Diverticula then result from the force exerted by the muscular layer. The force and pressure are lowest in the widest portion of the colon, the cecum, and highest in the narrowest portion, the sigmoid. Diverticula of the colon are most rare in those parts of the world where the diet of the inhabitants is very high in fiber, and we have already seen how fiber increases the bulk of the colonic content.

Can Diet Prevent the Development of Diverticula?

The current evidence is far from complete, but it certainly suggests that individuals raised on a diet high in fiber seem to have a much better chance of avoiding diverticula and their complications than people who consume a low-fiber diet. If we add to that the advantage of a high-fiber diet, simply in terms of reduction of coronary artery disease, obesity, and probably also the formation of cancers of the colon, this is enough good reason to adopt a high-fiber diet.

What Is the Point of Using a High-Fiber Diet if I Already Have Diverticulosis of the Colon?

Infection, perforation, and bleeding are the chief complications of diverticulitis, and it is not uncommon to develop an abscess in the wall of a sigmoid diverticulum. If you have never had diverticulitis, despite having the pouches known as diverticula, or even if you have completely recovered from an acute episode of diverticulitis, which fortunately did not require surgical intervention to cure it, then there is all the more reason to prevent further episodes by increasing the bulk of your diet.

Does a High-Fiber Diet Have a Place in the Management of an Acute Episode? No, a high-fiber diet is absolutely not recommended and can cause further trouble in the acute situation.

Recovery from an episode of acute diverticulitis may be slow, and you must gradually increase dietary fiber. When your physician feels that you have made a complete recovery, then slowly begin increasing the fiber in your diet, taking several weeks to reach the desired level of intake.

What Is the Ideal High-Fiber Diet?

Fiber is the nonabsorbable parts of fruits, vegetables, salads, grain cereals, and legumes (kidney beans, red lentils, soybeans), and we should have as our goal between 25 and 30 grams of fiber daily. Some individuals need more, others need less.

I find it useful for my patients to keep a food diary for three days so they can jot down their ordinary diet and calculate (from Table 3) the actual amount of fiber they are consuming. It requires no higher math, and it is well worth the investment of time. I urge them to begin slowly and stay with the diet.

How Long Do I Stay on This High-Fiber Diet to Control My Diverticula, and Does It Work?

One of my hopes in writing this book is that its readers will review their usual diet and aim at increasing their fiber for the many good reasons I have already outlined. If you have the added reason of curing a diseased colon, then my answer is that you should try to stay on the diet for life, or for as long as you can tolerate it.

I know of no controlled trials that prove conclusively that high fiber prevents diverticulosis in individuals, but I believe that it is reasonable to try and see if it prevents you from having another attack. You will have lost nothing and may even have improved other aspects of your health.

Is There any Relationship between the Irritable Bowel Syndrome (IBS) and Colonic Diverticula?

The finding of a few colonic diverticula in individuals suffering from the irritable bowel syndrome raises the question of whether the diseases are related. Diverticula are common in the general population and probably have little to do with the symptoms of irritable bowel syndrome, so you need not automatically switch to a high-fiber diet to cure irritable bowel symptoms. If, however, your irritable bowel syndrome includes a long history of constipation and dependence on laxatives, then the high-fiber approach may be helpful for you. If this diet causes you some discomfort while you are first adjusting to it, your physician may help you by prescribing an antispasmodic medication. This sometimes works. Taking a psyllium plant seed preparation, such as Metamucil®, can help during the transition period. In view of the widespread popularity of Metamucil among physicians and patients, we may very well wonder why it is not routinely prescribed to all individuals who have to increase their fiber intake. Although this substance is harmless, it is preferable to try to increase your dietary fiber before turning to other methods.

A Word on Jejunal Diverticulosis. An isolated diverticulum of the jejunum often discovered in the course of a routine gastrointestinal X-ray series with barium is actually of no significance. On occasion, however, an individual may suffer from weight loss, abdominal distention, fatty stools, and malabsorption, and will be discovered to have extensive diverticulosis of the small bowel, possibly resulting from a congenital condition. These pockets of the small bowel wall act as reservoirs for bacterial overgrowth to which the normal microbial inhabitants of the colon will migrate. It is one of the causes of malabsorption that results from bacterial overgrowth.

The primary approach to this condition is pharmacological since we cannot surgically remove all these diverticula. Thus we depend on suppressing or reducing the bacterial overgrowth with the appropriate antibiotics.

But there is a complementary role for diet therapy in this instance of malabsorption. The diet should be rich in carbohydrates and protein, and low in animal fat. However, starch and protein yield only about 4 calories per gram, whereas fat yields about 9 calories per gram. You can immediately see that you will have to increase your intake of carbohydrates and protein considerably if you are to gain or maintain your weight. There is another way of getting fat absorbed in this situation that does not require the usual, complex methods necessary to absorb the ordinary fat in our diet, which occurs by way of the long-chain fatty acids. Instead, if medium-chain triglycerides (MCT) are eaten, they can be absorbed directly into the portal blood vein of the abdomen. This oily material may be used in cooking or, easier still, simply taken by mouth. There are several various forms currently available. Mead-Johnson manufactures one called Portogen®, but this may contain lactose and be unsatisfactory for those who are intolerant of lactose, the sugar in milk. For these individuals, the MCT cooking oil is the better route.

To conclude this chapter: remember that our aim is to prevent the formation of colonic diverticula and to prevent the already-formed diverticula from progressing on to diverticulitis by the diligent continued use of a high-fiber diet. Remember, to get in the amount of fiber you need, your gut may experience some initial abdominal discomfort in going from a low- to a high-fiber diet. Patients may temporarily improve and are tempted to abandon the effort, but this is precisely the time to stay with the high-fiber intake. Keep a food diary, use Table 3 in this book to calculate your fiber intake, and stick to the high-fiber diet—it has long-term payoffs.

12

❋ ❋ ❋

WHAT SHOULD WE FEED THE INFLAMED INTESTINE? ULCERATIVE COLITIS AND CROHN'S DISEASE

We have already discussed the common functional disorder of the bowel—irritable bowel syndrome, or IBS as it is usually abbreviated. Now we need to turn our attention to the more serious inflammations of the bowel. They are mainly of two distinct groups: ulcerative colitis and Crohn's disease. They are grouped together as inflammatory bowel diseases, abbreviated IBD, and are not to be confused with IBS, irritable bowel syndrome.

Ulcerative colitis is an inflammation of unknown origin that can attack any or all parts of the large bowel or colon. If the whole colon is involved, it is called *universal ulcerative colitis*. If only a part is involved, a more specific label is used according to the area involved—for example, *sigmoid colitis*. The label for ulcerative colitis of the rectum is *ulcerative proctitis*.

Crohn's disease, on the other hand, is another different type of inflammation, which can occur anywhere along the intestinal tract, from the mouth to the rectum. It is seen most frequently

in the lower intestinal tract, the ileum (*ileitis*) or ileum and colon (*ileo colitis*). Its cause, like ulcerative colitis, is not known
at present.

The word *inflammation* comes from the Latin root *inflam-
mare* that means to set on fire and the part of the bowel that is
inflamed can be visualized as a burnt area.

Food is an area of discontent for most sufferers of gastrointestinal disorders, as well as their families. And there is a great
deal of disagreement about what diet is most beneficial in terms
of complementing other therapies. Our society places so much
emphasis on food, and the cultural climate is so preoccupied
with what is "natural" that we cannot help thinking about food.
Legend and folklore, plus deep psychic concerns about what
we ingest, reinforce all our instincts that food must play some
role in affecting the health of our intestinal tract. No wonder
my patients are troubled over whether their past dietary faults
have led to their present difficulties. Even more important, they
want to know what they should eat to get better, and get better
faster. I honestly believe that the expectations of some of my
patients are too high—diet and vitamins cannot cure in all
cases, but they do play a role in colitis and Crohn's disease.

For all my patients, I review what I consider the essentials
of a well-balanced, satisfactory, normal diet (Chapter 3). But
because some protein leaks from the inflamed intestinal lining,
people with these disorders must be sure they consume a diet
rich in protein. I also review the role of vitamins and trace minerals. Frankly, we have limited information on how inflammatory bowel disease is affected by food, in contrast to lactose
intolerance and gluten enteropathy, where we know so much.

IBD is a serious disorder and has important effects on the
gastrointestinal tract. And it carries with it the risk of lifelong
sensitivity or a recurrence of symptoms and pathological findings—even the risk of a cancerous development. But our information for the unfortunate sufferer on the role of diet in this
disease is fragmentary, meager, and unsatisfying.

We know that certain intestinal diseases are caused or influenced by too much of a particular type of food. Celiac disease in children is an excellent example. Eliminating one specific protein, gluten, from the diet stops this diarrheal disease. Doctors forbid wheat, rye, oats, and barley and insist parents and families read the labels on prepared foods. Unfortunately, it is not so simple in IBD. No one knows of any specific food the patient lacks or consumes too much of. So doctors sound permissive or unconcerned when they tell you to "eat whatever agrees with you." Some investigators have suggested the possibility that sugary breakfast cereals or a lack of grain or cereal in the diet might play a role in the early development of both ulcerative colitis and Crohn's disease, but few physicians and researchers are convinced of this hypothesis.

Smoking plays an interesting and important role in both these IBDs. Crohn's patients tend to be heavier smokers than the average individual without the disease. Ulcerative colitis patients smoke less. Even more striking is the well-established fact that some patients may have a flareup of their ulcerative colitis when they stop smoking. Does smoking really protect against ulcerative colitis? No one would really believe this, and I would not suggest a return to cigarette smoking as a method of treatment. Some preliminary studies have reported that nicotine patches improved some individuals, but the high degree of side effects render nicotine therapy, even for former smokers, a risky recommendation.

Caffeine and Alcohol

For many individuals, a cup of coffee, which contains 40 to 50 milligrams of caffeine, stimulates a bowel movement. (Although tea contains less *caffeine*, it has other substances of the same chemical family.) So it doesn't make sense to consume caffeine-containing beverages, including the cola family of drinks, if you are already having too many bowel movements, but I am not strict about this point.

Alcohol plays a large role in the social and business life of Western countries and is probably the most widely used tranquilizer. Moderate alcohol consumption is supposed to help the circulation, especially the circulation of the coronary arteries of the heart, and decrease certain negative components of the blood—the low-density lipoproteins (or LDLs)—which we have all read about in the media as a factor in heart disease. But alcohol has a deleterious effect on the subtle interplay of digestive enzymes that are released from the lining of the intestinal tract. When my patients are sick, I favor reducing or eliminating alcohol altogether, although I would not forbid some alcohol in the form of wine to stimulate the capricious appetite of an adult accustomed to drinking. When a patient with Crohn's disease is being treated with a drug called metronidazole (Flagyl®), alcohol is forbidden. A severe reaction may occur that resembles the effects of an alcoholic drink on someone who is being treated with Antabuse for alcoholism. This reaction can be serious and alarming.

A Dietary Approach to Ulcerative Colitis and Crohn's Disease

Nutrition does play an important part in recovery. The clearest case is the child with Crohn's disease or ulcerative colitis who is not growing because of the disease or the medications, especially steroids. Increasing the number of calories the child consumes leads to marked improvement, not only in weight but in growth and sexual development. For these children, nightly feedings of a liquid diet introduced through a tube into the nose has resulted in marked weight gain and general improvement in the patient's sense of well-being.

A well-balanced, nutritious diet is important for all of us, especially these sick people. They need a high-protein diet to make up for any lack of protein as well as to heal their intestinal walls: eggs, cheese, cereal, chicken, fish and meat, together with vegetables. But remember that a high-protein diet is a weight-reduction diet. The protein calories must be balanced by an increased amount of starches: potatoes, rice, pasta, bread, and cakes. Fats should not be automatically eliminated. Fat gives the body 9 calories for each gram of food eaten, whereas protein and starch give only 4. Since citrus fruits and salads are frequently cut back, vitamins, especially vitamin C, may be deficient (see section on vitamin supplements below). Foods should be reduced cautiously in the patient's diet because a great many patients have arbitrarily eliminated a great many desirable foods from their diets.

The questions I am most often asked have to do with lactose and dairy products, fiber (raw foods, salad, and cooked vegetables), and vitamin supplements. The important point to remember is that your past food experiences, your tolerance and tolerance of certain foods, must be taken into account. If your past history has shown a clear-cut intolerance for a specific food or a class of foods, discuss this with your doctor. You are not supposed to leave outside the consulting room what you have learned about yourself in the past—but be sure you are convinced not by one bad experience but by careful observation over a long time.

Lactose and Dairy Products

Patients and doctors for a long time have thought and wondered whether dairy products are bad for patients with IBD. Some have even suggested that patients weaned too early from breast milk or not breast fed may have a greater tendency to have colitis, but this notion has not stood up. Intolerance to lactose, the sugar of milk, is however, rather widespread in the general population, and this intolerance increases as we get older because the intestinal enzyme, lactase, which splits the molecule of lactose, diminishes with age. This leads to the undigested and unabsorbed lactose (milk sugar) getting into the lower intestine, where bacteria get to work on this material. Cramps, bloating, gas, and passage of loose, watery, and at times foul movements follow. Any extensive inflammation of the small intestine, where this enzyme is located says to me that there is not enough lactase to do the job. Small areas of inflammation are not important in this regard, and some people are intolerant of other elements in milk—the proteins (casein and lactalbumin).

By the time I get to see patients with ulcerative colitis and ileitis, most have already discovered whether dairy products make a difference—whether they increase the discomfort, lead to diarrhea and cramps, or in some cases even to increased blood in the stool. If considerable experience convinces me and my patients these can't be tolerated, then I advise avoiding them. To the patient with a past history of milk intolerance since childhood, to suggest a trial with a low-lactose diet is beside the point. I have not found that testing the patient with a lactose tolerance test helps. Instead, the ability of the patient to tolerate dairy products in the course of real life is much more useful. If there really is lactose intolerance, the patient should avoid milk, cheese, ice cream, and butter only. I am not convinced that lactose incorporated into prepared foods is important, but I advise patients to read the label on food for the lactose content. For those on a low-lactose diet, there is no substitute for cheese and most ice cream, although lactose-free ice cream is beginning to appear commercially. Some margarines contain milk solids, so here too one must read the labels. For milk, non-dairy creamers can be substituted.

If this ritual has not had a clear-cut effect in two weeks, I abandon it and suggest a gradual intake of milk. If after this dietary trial you and your doctor have a feeling that it is useful, you might consider the use of a commercially available lactase-treated milk (Lactaid®, for example) to see whether this treated milk is tolerated and worth the effort. In some patients, intolerance may not be an all or nothing matter. You might be tolerant of a small amount (less than 8 ounces) of a product, but with any more of this product, your symptoms might return.

The downside of the low-lactose diet should be considered:

it reduces calcium intake. (A reduction of calcium in the diet is discussed in detail in Chapter 3.) It is difficult to get enough calcium into our diet if we eliminate most milk products. Calcium supplements fortified with vitamin D become necessary to prevent deficiency of calcium, especially in pregnant women, women after childbirth, postmenopausal women, and patients receiving steroids, since steroids may have a weakening effect on the bones.

Fiber

Nowadays everyone knows that we ought to have a good intake of fresh fruits and vegetables, as well as grains, because our Western diet is too refined. Everyone has read over and over again in the popular press that in certain parts of the world (Africa) where people eat lots of roots and fibers the population does not suffer from any of the intestinal disorders we have in the developed world—spastic colon, irritable colon, constipation, diverticulitis, and cancer of the colon. This is true, but it would be simpleminded to believe that this is due only to the high fiber in these populations. These countries may not have the environmental pollution we have, food additives are probably nonexistent, and there's no IRS or other stressors. But be that as it may, a diet adequate in fiber is a healthy one.

However healthy this kind of diet may be in general, when you are sick with diarrhea and have abdominal cramps and active bleeding, it makes no sense to maintain a high intake of raw fruits and vegetables. At these times, the diet should contain cooked vegetables and canned fruits. Bananas are easily tolerated when they are ripe. For steamed vegetables, I would skip the cabbage family (cabbage, brussels sprouts, broccoli, and cauliflower, though I have been told by patients that the florets of broccoli seem to be well tolerated). Potatoes and whole grain breads provide some fiber as well. In those of you who can tolerate them, and only through trial and error can you tell, limited amounts of fresh fruits and vegetables can be eaten, unless there is an area in the intestine that has been narrowed by a previous inflammation and a tight scar. In this instance, it would be foolhardy to run the risk of blocking such a narrowed area and becoming completely obstructed. I have seen such scarred areas become blocked by corn on the cob, as well as tough, stringy vegetables, popcorn, and even by a number of pimento-stuffed jumbo olives! A strict low residue diet is given in Table 11.

Vitamin Supplements

Patients, their parents, their family, and doctors are overwhelmed by a flood of media stories on the role of diet and vitamins in treating IBD. What do we know that makes sense and what supplements are recommended? With a patient eating three, well-balanced meals, the problem depends on whether he or she is digesting and absorbing the elements of the food properly. There is always some doubt about this in patients with ileitis and colitis. It makes sense to supplement the normal diet in these cases with a standard brand of multivitamins. Since fresh fruits and vegetables as well as fruit juices are often the first to be eliminated from the patient's diet, vitamin C (ascorbic acid) supplements are in order. Because dairy products are routinely reduced or eliminated, lack of calcium may result. To make up for this deficiency, be sure the calcium supplement you take is not in the form of calcium lactate—which defeats the purpose of reducing lactate in the diet.

For the patient who becomes anemic (who has low hemoglobin in the blood and a low red-cell count), the condition may have developed for several reasons: rectal bleeding, inadequate intakes of iron and the blood-forming vitamins folic acid and vitamin B12, failure to absorb vitamin B12 in the ileum, failure to absorb iron in the duodenum, or the use of a particular drug that interferes with the absorption of folic acid, such as sulfasalazine, which is often used to treat IBD. Your doctor can easily check the blood levels of vitamin B12, folate (folic acid), and iron. Based on these tests, vitamin B12 can be given by injection

Table 11. Low Residue Diet

The low residue diet is used for patients with intestinal disturbances and for pre- and postoperative cases. This diet restricts the intake of dietary fiber and of milk which has medium residue. If the purpose of the diet is only to reduce the amount of residue in the lower bowel and to decrease fecal output, milk and milk products are not restricted. Highly seasoned and fried foods are generally omitted but individual tolerances should be considered. Foods should be well chewed and meals should be eaten slowly. Dietary fiber is reduced by using refined cereal grains, certain whole, well-cooked tender vegetables, cooked or canned fruits (without any seeds or skins), and tender meats.

Adequacy: The low residue diet is planned to meet the Recommended Daily Dietary Allowances.

Food Groups	Foods Allowed	Foods Not Allowed
Milk Group (2 cups daily)	Limit to two cups daily, whole, low-fat, skim, or buttermilk, pasteurized eggnog, and yogurt	Milk and milk beverages in excess of 2 cups per day
Meat Group (2 servings daily) **Meat, Poultry, or Fish**	Broiled, baked, or boiled beef, lean pork, lamb, liver, poultry, fish, salmon, tuna	Fried, smoked, barbecued, or spicy meats, fat pork, luncheon meats, frankfurters, sausage, poultry, skin
Meat Substitutes	Eggs, cottage cheese, cream cheese, milk, cheddar or American cheese, smooth peanut butter	Fried eggs, sharp cheese, crunchy peanut butter, and dried beans, peas, or lentils

(*continued*)

Table 11. Low Residue Diet (continued)

Food Groups	Foods Allowed	Foods Not Allowed
Vegetable and Fruit Group (4 servings daily)		
Potato Substitute	White potato, white rice, noodles, macaroni and spaghetti	Fried potatoes, potato or corn chips, potato skin, brown rice
Vegetables	Canned or cooked mild-flavored vegetables (without seeds or coarse fiber)—beets, carrots, mushrooms, peas, green or wax beans, pumpkin, spinach, squash; pureed (strained) vegetable, vegetable juice	All raw vegetables, strongly flavored, coarse vegetables, and those with seeds
Fruits	Canned or cooked fruits—apples, cherries, peaches, pears, apricots, or grapes (without seeds or skins); fresh fruit (without skin, seeds, or rough fiber)—banana, orange, or grapefruit sections (without membrane); pureed (strained) fruit, fruit juice	Raw fruits other than those listed, dried fruits, fruits with rough skins or seeds—raw apples, berries, dates, figs, fresh grapes, plums, prunes, and raisins

(continued)

Table 11. **Low Residue Diet** (continued)

Food Groups	Foods Allowed	Foods Not Allowed
Soups	Broth, bouillon, strained vegetable soup, strained cream soups (use milk allowance); soups made with allowed meats and vegetables	Highly seasoned soups, soups made with ingredients which are not allowed
Bread and Cereal Group (4 servings daily)	Enriched white bread, plain rolls, Saltines or soda crackers, melba toast	Breads or crackers made with whole-grain flour, bran, or containing seeds or cracked wheat
Cereals	Refined cooked cereals such as cream of wheat, cream of rice, grits; processed ready-to-eat cereals such as cornflakes, puffed rice, puffed wheat, plain rice cereals	Whole grain or bran cereals, granola
Miscellaneous Fats	Butter, margarine, cream, mayonnaise, vegetable oil, shortening	Salt pork, lard, nuts

to avoid the problem of absorption. Folic acid can be taken in pill form and iron can be replaced either by tablets or, if need be, in exceptional cases, by injection. In my experience many patients with IBD have abdominal distress if they take iron by mouth, especially cramps and constipation. Their stool may turn black and be confused with rectal blood. It may be necessary to try a few preparations of iron before finding one that agrees with you.

What Is the Role of Trace Elements?

Several vital substances circulate in the blood in very small amounts. Called "trace elements," these substances are essential for the healthy functioning of the body's tissues.

The trace element we know most about is *zinc.* Researchers have found that some patients with skin and mouth problems, as well as intestinal problems, may have low stores of zinc. These patients have been nutritionally deprived through failure to absorb this substance or by starvation, given inadequate food, or intravenous fluids that lack the proper amount of zinc. For these patients, zinc should be given in a pill form.

Another trace element, *selenium,* can cause heart trouble if it is absent from the diet, but it is a rare deficiency. It is usually seen in individuals who receive all their nutrition intravenously, a procedure called *total parenteral hyperalimentation* (TPN). This deficiency has now been corrected by including selenium in all TPN solutions given to sick patients.

Food Supplements

Because patients with IBD may have a capricious appetite or because of poor eating, some individuals may be given food supplements to increase both calories and nutrients. Some of these fluid preparations are high in calories and pleasantly flavored, but they are meant as supplements, not as replacements for real food—not unless there is a mechanical blockage that prevents food from passing through the gut. Ensure®, Sustical®, or Flexi-Cal®, are among the popular brand-name supplements you may be prescribed. The limitations in other "elemental diets," as they are called, are their expense and unpalatable flavors. Patients are not happy to take them.

Another way of increasing calories—even in patients who have had some of the intestine removed or in those with an inflamed bowel—is to give them fat in a form that does not require the formation of micelles by bile salts and pancreatic juice which occur normally in digestion. What we give these patients is fat in the form of medium-chain triglycerides (MCTs), which are shorter chains of fatty acid than we find in our normal diets. Corn oil, for example, is a long-chain fatty acid, but is not easily absorbed. The medium-chain triglycerides are digestible and are described at length in Chapter 7 on malabsorption.

Enteral Nutrition

This term means supplying the patient's nutrition by mouth in a liquid form that can be easily absorbed by the small intestine. With this approach, the diet is reduced to its essential chemical elements, a procedure recommended especially by our British colleagues in the treatment of Crohn's disease. In some studies, elemental diets taken by mouth have reduced the complications of Crohn's disease of the intestine.

These elemental diet preparations contain the smallest elements of the diets—amino acids, sugar, triglycerides or fatty acids, vitamins, and trace elements. It is difficult to persuade patients with Crohn's disease to take adequate amounts of these preparations because they are often so unpalatable. Even the astronauts rebelled against taking the elemental diet. But elemental enteral diets do appear to have a place in acute ulcerative colitis before surgery or as a way of treating inflammation in Crohn's disease.

Prevention of Oxalate Kidney Stones

At first glance, the title of this section may seem far afield from the dietary approaches we have been considering in this chapter. But patients with inflammatory bowel disease (IBD), both Crohn's and ulcerative colitis, can and do often suffer from kidney stones, some of which are oxalate kidney stones. So it is important for us to understand how intestinal disease can contribute to the formation of oxalate stones.

What is oxalate, and how does the intestinal inflammation lead to problems? In this series of questions and answers, I have followed the extremely useful small book entitled *The Low Oxalate Diet Book for the Prevention of Oxalate Kidney Stones*, largely the work of Dr. Alan Hoffman and his colleagues, Denise Nye, Cheryl Fischer, and Mary Stublefield, published by the Clinical Center of the University of California Medical School at San Diego Medical Center, with their permission and encouragement.

Oxalate, which is the same as oxalic acid, is an organic compound that occurs naturally in food, especially in foods of plant origin. It is not essential for life and is excreted in the urine.

What are the foods that contain the high amounts of oxalate? The highest concentrations are found in green leafy vegetables, beans, cereals, beets, rhubarb, chocolate, tea, coffee, and peanuts.

What happens when oxalate is eaten by normal people? The ordinary diet contains between 80 and 100 milligrams of oxalate a day, and in most people, it is not absorbed, but forms insoluble calcium salts in the small intestine, which are excreted in the stool. In hyperoxaluria, on the other hand, excessive amounts of oxalate are excreted in the urine, and this leads to stones. For most individuals, an increased amount of oxalate in the urine stems from an increased absorption of the oxalate eaten.

How does the increased absorption take place in individuals with intestinal disease whose small intestine has been affected by disease or surgery, or by bypass surgery? Two mechanisms seem to be very important. First, patients with small bowel disease absorb fatty acids poorly. Calcium in the intestine forms soaps with the fatty acids rather than with the oxalate. The oxalate thus remains in solution, allowing for increased absorption. Moreover, patients with intestinal disease, especially if the ileum is affected, have trouble absorbing their bile salts. That results in the passage of bile salts into the colon, which normally functions to absorb water and solidify the feces. The presence of increased bile salts in the colon enhances the absorption of oxalate in the colon.

What is the best way to prevent the formation of oxalate stones? You must restrict your oxalate intake in the diet, limit your fat intake, increase fluid each day to dilute the urine of its oxalate contents, and avoid vitamin C supplements. This last point is important since vitamin C is converted into oxalate in the body of some individuals.

If your kidneys function normally, then you can supplement your diet with calcium in the form of calcium gluconate or calcium carbonate, which can block the absorption of oxalate. For some individuals, aluminum hydroxide will also block the absorption of oxalate, but not as effectively as calcium.

Rich fatty foods should be avoided, particularly butter, margarine, fried foods, and rich creams and sauces. On the other hand, cereals, meat, and some dietary products are low in oxalate. See the table that follows (Table 12) for the oxalate content of many foods and a low-oxalate meal plan. Your goal should be to eat no more than 40 to 50 milligrams of oxalate a day.

Table 12. Foods to Avoid: These Foods Are High in Oxalate (more than 15 mg oxalate per serving)

Vegetables	Fruits	Beverages	Miscellaneous
Beans in tomato sauce	Berries black	Beer, lager Tuborg Pilsner	Chocolate Cocoa
Beets	blue	Ovaltine	Grits
Celery	green goose	(24 mg/8 oz.)	(white corn)
Chard, Swiss	raspberries	Tea (132–181.2	Peanuts
Collards	black	mg/8 oz.)	Pecans
Dandelion greens	Currants, red		Soybean
Eggplant	Grapes,		crackers
Escarole	Concord		Wheat germ
Leek	Lemon peel		
Okra	Lime peel		
Parsley	Rhubarb		
Pepper, green			
Pokeweed			
Potatoes, sweet			
Rutabagas			
Spinach			
Squash, summer			

Foods to Use: These Foods Contain Small Amounts of Oxalate
(0–2 mg oxalate per serving)

Vegetables	Fruits	Beverages	Miscellaneous
Broccoli	Avocado	Apple juice	Butter
Brussels	Banana	Barley water	Cheese, cheddar
sprouts	Cheries	Beer, bottled	Chicken noodle soup
Cabbage	Grapes, Thompson	Cider	Cornflakes
Cauliflower	seedless	Coca-Cola	Eggs
Chive	Mangoes	Grapfruit juice	Egg noodles (Chow Mein)
Cucumber	Melons	Lemon squash drink	Fish (except sardines)
Lettuce	Nectarines	(lemonade)	Jelly with allowed fruit
Mushrooms	Peaches	Lucozade, bottled	Lemon juice
Peas	canned	Milk	Lime juice
Potatoes, white	Hiley	Orange juice	Macaroni
Radishes	Srokes	Pepsi-Cola	Margarine
Rice	Pineapple	Pineapple juice	Meats
Turnips	Plums	Sherry, dry	Oatmeal, porridge
	Golden Gage	Wine	Oxtail soup
	Green Gage		Poultry
			Red plum jam

(continued)

Oxalate Content by Food Groups

	Oxalate mg/100 gm
Cereal and Cereal Products	
Bread, white	4.9
Cake, fruit	11.8
Cake, sponge	7.4
Cornflakes	2.0
Crackers, soybean	207.0
Egg noodle (Chow Mein)	1.0
Grits (white corn)	41.0
Macaroni, boiled	1.0
Oatmeal, porridge	1.0
Spaghetti in tomato sauce	4.0
Wheat germ	269.0
Milk and Milk Products	
Butter	0.0
Cheese, cheddar	0.0
Margarine	0.0
Milk	0.15
Meats and Eggs	
Bacon, streaky fried	3.3
Beef, canned corned	0.0
Beef, topside roast	0.0
Chicken, roast	0.0
Eggs, boiled	0.0
Fish	
haddock	0.2
plaice	0.3
sardines	4.8
Ham	1.6
Hamburger, grilled	0.0
Lamb, roast	trace
Liver	7.1
Pork, roast	1.7
Vegetables	
Asparagus	5.2
Beans, green boiled	15.0
Beans in tomato sauce	19.0
Beetroot, boiled	675.0
Beetroot, pickled	500.0
Broccoli, boiled	trace

Oxalate Content by Food Groups (continued)

	Oxalate mg/100 gm
Vegetables (continued)	
Brussels sprouts, boiled	0.0
Cabbage, boiled	0.0
Carrots, canned	4.0
Cauliflower, boiled	1.0
Celery	20.0
Chard, Swiss	645.0
Chive	1.1
Collards	74.0
Corn, yellow	5.2
Cucumber, raw	1.0
Dandelion greens	24.6
Eggplant	18.0
Escarole	31.0
Kale	13.0
Leek	89.0
Lettuce	3.0
Lima beans	4.3
Mushrooms	2.0
Mustard greens	7.7
Okra	146.0
Onion, boiled	3.0
Parsley, raw	100.0
Parsnips	10.0
Peas, canned	1.0
Pepper, green	16.0
Pokeweed	475.0
Potatoes, white boiled	0.0
Potatoes, sweet	56.0
Radishes	0.3
Rice, boiled	0.0
Rutabagas	19.0
Spinach, boiled	750.0
Spinach, frozen	600.0
Squash, summer	22.0
Tomatoes, raw	2.0
Turnips, boiled	1.0
Watercress, early fine curled	10.0

(*continued*)

	Oxalate mg/100 gm
Fruits	
Apples, raw	3.0
Apricots	2.8
Avocado	0.0
Banana, raw	trace
Berries	
black	18.0
blue	15.0
dew	14.0
green goose	88.0
raspberries, black	53.0
raspberries, red	15.0
strawberries, canned	15.0
strawberries, raw	10.0
Cherries	
bing	0.0
sour	1.1
Currants	
black	4.3
red	19.0
Fruit salad, canned	12.0
Grapes	
concord	25.0
Thompson seedless	0.0
Lemon peel	83.0
Lime peel	110.0
Mangoes	0.0
Melons	
cantaloupe	0.0
casaba	0.0
honeydew	0.0
watermelon	0.0
Nectarines	0.0
Oranges, raw	4.0
Peaches	
Alberta	5.0
canned	1.2
Hiley	0.0
Stokes	1.2

	Oxalate mg/100 gm
Fruits (continued)	
Pears	
Bartlett, canned	1.7
Pineapple, canned	1.0
Plums	
Damson	10.0
Golden Gage	1.1
Green Gage	0.0
Preserves	
red plum jam	0.5
strawberry jam	9.4
Prunes, Italian	5.8
Rhubarb	
canned	600.0
stewed, no sugar	860.0
Nuts	
Peanuts, roasted	187.0
Pecans	202.0
Confectionary	
Chocolate, plain	117.0
Jelly, with allowed fruit	0.0
Marmalade	10.8
Plain candies	0.0
Beverages, nonalcoholic	
Barley water, bottled	0.0
Coca-Cola	trace
Coffee (0.5 g Nescafe/100 ml)	3.2
Lemon squash drink (lemonade)	1.0
Lucozade, bottled (soda)	0.0
Orange squash drink (orangeade)	2.5
Ovaltine drink, 2 gm in 100 ml	10.0
Pepsi-Cola	trace
Ribena, concentrate (black currant drink)	2.0
Tea, Indian	
2 min. infusion	55.0
4 min. infusion	72.0
6 min. infusion	78.0
Tea, rosehip	4.0

(*continued*)

Oxalate Content by Food Groups (continued)

	Oxalate mg/100 gm
Juices	
Apple juice	trace
Cranberry juice	6.6
Grape juice	5.8
Grapefruit juice	0.0
Orange juice	0.5
Pineapple juice	0.0
Tomato juice	5.0
Beverages, alcoholic	
Beer	
bottled	0.0
draft	1.0
lager draft, Tuborg Pilsner	4.0
Stout, Guinness draft	2.0
Cider	0.0
Sherry, dry	trace
Wine	
port	trace
rosé	1.5
white	0.0
Miscellaneous	
Cocoa, dry powder	623.0
Coffee powder (Nescafe)	33.0
Chicken noodle soup	1.0
Lemon juice	1.0
Lime juice	0.0
Ovaltine, powder canned	35.0
Oxtail soup	1.0
Pepper	419.0
Tomato soup	3.0
Vegetable soup	5.0

100 grams = ½ cup, usually

Low-Oxalate Meal Plan (40–50 mg)

Foods	Little or No Oxalate (less than 2 mg oxalate per serving; eat as desired)	Moderate Oxalate Content (2–10 mg oxalate per serving; limit to two 1/2 cup servings a day)	High Oxalate Foods (more than 10 mg oxalate per serving; avoid completely if possible)
Beverages/Juices	Apple juice Beer, bottled Coca-Cola (12 oz. limit/day) Distilled alcohol Grapefruit juice Lemonade or limeade w/o peel Wine, red, rosé Pepsi-Cola (12 oz. limit/day) Pineapple juice Tap water (preferred for extra calcium)	Coffee, any kind (8 oz. serving) Cranberry juice (4 oz.) Grape juice (4 oz.) Orange juice (4 oz.) Tomato juice (4 oz.) Nescafe powder	Draft Stout, Guinness draft Lager, Tuborg Pilsner Juices containing berries not allowed Ovaltine and other mixed beverage mixes Tea, cocoa

(continued)

Low-Oxalate Meal Plan (40–50 mg) (continued)

Foods	Little or No Oxalate (less than 2 mg oxalate per serving; eat as desired)	Moderate Oxalate Content (2–10 mg oxalate per serving; limit to two 1/2 cup servings a day)	High Oxalate Foods (more than 10 mg oxalate per serving; avoid completely if possible)
Milk (2 or more cups)	Buttermilk Low-fat milk Low-fat yogurt with allowed fruit Skim milk		
Meat Group	Eggs Cheese, cheddar Lean lamb, beef, or pork Poultry Seafood	Sardines	Baked beans canned in tomato sauce Peanut butter Soybean curd (Tofu)
Vegetables	Avocado Brussels sprouts Cabbage Cauliflower Mushrooms Onions Peas, green Potatoes (Irish) Radishes	Asparagus Broccoli Carrots Corn sweet white sweet yellow Cucumber, peeled Green peas, canned Lettuce, iceberg	Beans green wax dried Beets tops root greens

Foods	Little or No Oxalate (less than 2 mg oxalate per serving; eat as desired)	Moderate Oxalate Content (2–10 mg oxalate per serving; limit to two ½ cup servings a day)	High Oxalate Foods (more than 10 mg oxalate per serving; avoid completely if possible)
Vegetables (continued)		Lima beans	Celery
		Parsnips	Chard, Swiss
		Tomato, 1 small	Chive
		Turnips	Collards
			Dandelion greens
			Eggplant
			Escarole
			Kale
			Leeks
			Mustard greens
			Okra
			Parsley
			Peppers, green
			Pokeweed
			Potatoes, sweet
			Rutabagas
			Spinach
			Summer squash
			Watercress

(continued)

Low-Oxalate Meal Plan (40–50 mg) (continued)

Foods	Little or No Oxalate (less than 2 mg oxalate per serving; eat as desired)	Moderate Oxalate Content (2–10 mg oxalate per serving; limit to two 1/2 cup servings a day)	High Oxalate Foods (more than 10 mg oxalate per serving; avoid completely if possible)
Fruits	Avocado	Apple	Blackberries
	Banana	Apricots	Blueberries
	Cherries, bing	Black currants	Concord grapes
	Grapefruit	Cherries, red sour	Red currants
	Grapes, Thompson	Orange, edible portion	Dewberries
	seedless	Peaches, Alberta	Fruit cocktail
	Mangoes	Pears	Gooseberries
	Melons	Pineapple	Lemon peel
	cantaloupe	Plums, Damson	Lime peel
	casaba	Prunes, Italian	Orange peel
	honeydew		Raspberries
	watermelon		Rhubarb
	Nectarines		Strawberries
	Peaches, Hiley		Tangerine
	Plums, green or Golden		
	Age		

Foods	Little or No Oxalate (less than 2 mg oxalate per serving; eat as desired)	Moderate Oxalate Content (2–10 mg oxalate per serving; limit to two 1/2 cup servings a day)	High Oxalate Foods (more than 10 mg oxalate per serving; avoid completely if possible)
Bread/Starches	Cornflakes Macaroni Noodles Oatmeal Rice Spaghetti White bread	Cornbread Sponge cake Spaghetti, canned in tomato sauce	Fruit cake Grits, white corn Soybean crackers Wheat germ
Fats and Oils	Bacon Mayonnaise Salad dressing Vegetable oils		Nuts peanuts pecans
Miscellaneous	Jelly or preserves (made with allowed fruits) Lemon, lime juice Salt, pepper (1 tsp/day) Soups with ingredients allowed Sugar	Chicken noodle soup, dehydrated	Chocolate, cocoa Pepper (in excess of 1 tsp/day) Vegetable soup Tomato soup

13

* * *

CANCER OF
THE COLON
AND RECTUM

Cancer of the colon and rectum (colorectal cancer) is a first-class world problem, especially in areas of North America and Europe and other industrialized countries where lifestyle and diet have been pointed to as causes of the rise in the incidence of this cancer. The rising incidence of colorectal cancer is front-page news in our newspapers and journals. It is the third most common cancer in the United States, just below breast and lung cancer. It has been reported that in 1991 there were approximately 160,000 new cases in the United States and 60,000 deaths related to this malignancy, secondary only to lung cancer. Throughout the world, it is the third most common cancer in men and the fourth most common in women.

For all these reasons, especially the rising rate of this cancer, anything we might possibly do to prevent this disease is worth considering carefully. Surgical removal of the tumor and the use of adjunctive chemotherapy or radiotherapy are our only realistic methods of treatment at present. If a dietary program can do any good, it must be as prevention. Diet therapy has no real place in the treatment of an already established cancer of the colon and rectum.

What Does the Study of the Incidence and Occurrence of Cancer Throughout the World Tell Us about This Disease?

The frequency of colon cancer varies greatly among different populations. The highest rates are in the Westernized areas of North America, Australia, and New Zealand, with slightly lower rates in Europe. The lowest rates occur in Asia, South America, and Africa.

The difference between these areas is remarkable. Colon cancer in males is sixty times more frequent in the high-rate areas compared with the low-rate areas. Rectal cancer is twenty times higher in males in the high-risk areas compared with low-risk areas. The incidence in the United States has been increasing for cancer of the colon, but not for rectal carcinoma. Both colon and rectal cancer rates have risen in nonwhite people in the United States during the same period (since 1950). The striking feature of these studies is that the risk of colorectal cancer rises rapidly in populations moving from low-risk to high-risk areas. This has been dramatically confirmed in Japanese populations who have migrated to Hawaii or the continental United States.

While an individual's genes may confer susceptibility to colorectal cancer, dietary studies reveal that different lifestyles play a dramatic role in the development of colorectal cancer. Among the first changes in lifestyle that people experience as they reach new areas is the *change in diet*. Because of the strong circumstantial evidence for a link between diet and colorectal cancer, much research and thought have concentrated on this area of prevention.

What Is Known about the Links between Diet and Colorectal Cancer?

Fats

Several pieces of information suggest that diets high in fat pre-dispose an individual to colorectal cancer. The cancer rates are higher in people with a high total intake of fat and lower in those eating less fat.

On the average, despite the public warning of health offi-cials, fat—for instance, saturated and unsaturated fat—con-tributes 40 to 45 percent of the calories consumed in the Western world, whereas fat accounts for only 10 to 15 percent of dietary calories in the low-risk populations of the world. In a study done in 1990, when the relationship between meat, fat, and fiber among a very large number (many thousands) of women was investigated, the result indicated that the risk of colon cancer increased with increasing levels of fat eaten. For example, the ratio of red meat to chicken, where red meat has the higher content of fat, corresponds to the incidence of co-lon cancer—in other words, the higher rate of cancer is asso-ciated with a higher consumption of red meat. The relationship of cancer and cholesterol seems to be associated with blood levels of cholesterol, but not all investigators agree on this point.

Experimental studies in animals also find a relationship be-tween high-fat diets and cancer of the colon. But fatty acids derived from polyunsaturated fish oils (omega-3 fatty acids) and monounsaturated olive oil pose less of a cancer threat to ani-mals.

Fiber

Studies in humans and animals suggest that dietary fiber may actually protect against the development of colon cancer. High-fiber diets, no matter how we define them (I have given some definitions in Chapter 3), could be correlated with lower levels of colon cancer. Much evidence supports this observation, but does not tell us about the importance of vegetables, fruits, nutrients, and micronutrients.

Fiber clearly increases the stool bulk. But what else can it tell us? In explaining the difference between the evidence of colon cancer in the population with the same or similar fat consumption, fiber seems to be an important protective factor. Increased fiber in the form of whole wheat and rye bread also appears helpful in contributing to fiber's benefits.

Foods That May Contribute to Colon Cancer

A group of substances in the colon are synthesized by the colonic bacteria and have the ability to cause genetic alterations in the bacteria of the colon. These so-called mutagenic substances may also play a role in cancer formation. Charcoal-broiled meats and fish, and to a lesser extent fried foods, may produce certain powerful mutagenic substances. A relationship between rectal cancer and the consumption of beer and ale has also been reported in at least two studies, a finding which needs further verification.

Vitamins and Trace Elements

Some incomplete studies suggest that carotene (beta-carotene or vitamin A) and vitamin C could act as antioxidants to prevent the formation of cancer. Selenium salts, vitamin E, and yellow vegetables or vegetables of the group known as the green cruciferous vegetables may also be involved, but the link between cancer and these factors remains unproven.

Calcium

The case of the role of calcium in preventing colorectal cancer is circumstantial, but the evidence is mounting. Researchers have suggested that the protective effect of calcium comes from its effect on the growth of precancerous and cancerous cells in the colon. The turnover of colonic abnormal cells can be reduced after supplemental levels of calcium are given to individuals with a family history of hereditary colon cancer, but no symptoms of colon cancer. For the present, the case for calcium as a protection against cancer is growing but has yet to be fully established.

What Can We Say about the Likelihood of All These Factors in Favor of Decreasing the Risk of Cancer of the Colon and Rectum?

We might formulate the answers as follows:

Probably related to cancer:

- High-fat and low-fiber intake, with the proviso that not all fats and all fat components are involved

Possibly related to cancer:

- Beer and ale consumption, especially for rectal cancer
- Low dietary selenium
- By-products of charcoal-broiled and fried meats and fish

What protects against cancer?

Probably protective against cancer:
- High-fiber diet

Possibly protective against cancer:
- Yellow vegetables, cruciferous vegetables, calcium, foods rich in vitamins A, C, and E

Given the Present State of Our Incomplete Knowledge, What Should I Do?

Aim for a diet low in fat—a good habit we have been discussing throughout the chapters. This means restricting your fat to less than 30 percent of your overall calories and probably 20 percent is closer to the ideal. See that you obtain at least 30 grams of fiber daily, including some whole wheat bread. Make sure your vegetables include some of the yellow and green vegetables— especially the cruciferous family—each day. If you are a woman, take 1.5 grams of calcium, and if need be, add a calcium supplement.

If you have a family history, including first-degree relations with cancer, premalignant polyps, or cancer, or have a premalignant case of polyps, in addition to regular medical checkups take a vitamin supplement that includes A, C, E, and selenium.

Preservatives, Sulforaphane, and Anti-Cancer Agents

Interestingly, some researchers have found that two widely used food preservatives increase levels of a natural cancer fighter in laboratory animals—and apparently do the same in humans. While advocates of natural foods doggedly object to the use of preservatives, others have found that the preservatives BHA and BHT stimulated the genes or the enzymes that destroy carcinogens before they form tumors. BHA and BHT are additives used as preservatives in cookies, crackers, and a wide variety of other foods. This does not mean that these additives should be increased, but they are important because they point out that there is a cancer-preventing mechanism that appears to be part of the explanation for the well-known anti-cancer properties of broccoli, cauliflower, brussels sprouts, and other members of the cruciferous family.

Some researchers say these are amazing vegetables, containing an amazing array of anti-cancer compounds. Most of the research on these vegetables has been done on animals, but some of it seems to be true for humans. The anti-cancer agent recently isolated from broccoli is *sulforaphane*, and it exerts its action in the same way as BHA and BHT—by working on a specific enzyme system in the tissues. While it is going to take the researchers a long time to figure out the mechanisms involved, as Dr. Walter Willett of the Harvard School of Public Health says, "This doesn't mean you can't do anything. You can eat more fruits and vegetables." One of the problems is that many people avoid the foods with the most potent anti-cancer properties. These include not only broccoli, but brussels sprouts and cauliflower, the so-called cruciferous vegetables. Others in this family are kale and cabbage. But the vegetables rich in folic acid (folate) also contain anti-cancer properties; these vegetables include spinach and collards.

Vitamins A and E—Should I Take Antioxidants?

Epidemiological studies on the relationships between antioxidants in the diet and cancer incidence have suggested that an increased level of vitamin E and beta-carotene (vitamin A) can reduce the mortality from cancer of the lung and colon. While one study questioned the role of vitamin A in smokers with lung cancer, this single study does not negate the many results of published studies. The antioxidant defenses in the body consist of many components of a variety of different molecular weights, and it may be that a fine balance between several antioxidants will be more important for the overall protective capacity of the system than the activity of a single substance. So we must assume there is some question mark about the role of a single antioxidant and the formation of human tumors. A lot more study is needed in this regard, but it would still seem prudent to have a diet that is rich in antioxidants.

Dietary Risk Factors in Colorectal Polyps:
Men and Women

Evidence continues to support the hypothesis that diet plays an important role as a risk factor in cancer of the colon. Most studies have been done on men; but some recent reports include women as well. For men, based on studies of polyps—the precursors of cancer of the colon—there is an increased risk for those who consume a diet high in saturated fats and low in dietary fiber. In another study, on polyps and diet in males, increased calorie intake was the risk factor for new or recurrent polyps.

In women, the development and recurrence of adematous polyps—the common form of polyps that develops into cancer—are associated with an increased intake of dietary saturated fats, an increased intake of meat in the diet, and a rise in the red meat-to-chicken ratio. It was also demonstrated that total fat played a role, but this risk is reduced if the individual's fiber intake is high.

From the material assembled in this chapter, you can see that, while the oncogenes (the genetic material) stimulate cancer and polyp formation, diet too may play a part in protecting against these tumors.

If you can't choose your genes, you can at least choose your foods.

Condensed to a formula: eat a high-fiber, low-fat diet, containing fruits and vegetables, especially yellows ones and the green, crunchy ones of the cabbage, broccoli family. Supplement your food intake with some calcium pills, and dietary supplements of vitamins C and E, along with beta-carotene (precursor of vitamin A). It will be good for you, in general, and may help in preventing the development of colonic polyps and colonic cancer.

14

* * *

INTESTINAL GAS

Many of the intestinal discomforts we complain about we blame on "gas." We pass gas from either end of the gastrointestinal tract—we belch it out or pass gas through the rectum. At times, we feel bloated and distended, and blame our symptoms on gas we cannot get rid of. We feel we are unable to pass or "break wind." We complain we are embarrassed by passing gas in social situations. There is an old, four-letter, Anglo-Saxon word for this, but physicians use the more neutral term *flatulence*.

The basic problem is that we don't know enough about the entire process of gas accumulation in the intestine and its passage along the alimentary canal. What we do know is based on one researcher, the ingenious medical investigator, Dr. Michael Levitt, who devised methods for the collection, measurement, and analysis of components of gas in the intestine.

Where Does This Gas Come From?

Some things about gas we do know. If we eat and talk, especially if we swallow rapidly or gulp our food, we accumulate air in the upper stomach. If we smoke a pipe or keep a cigar in our mouth for long periods of time or take deep drags of cigarettes, we can understand how air can be trapped in the gullet or the stomach. Certain foods are notoriously "gassy"—beans and members of the cabbage family.

There are three sources of gas formation in the gut.

1. Air swallowing is the major source of gas in the stomach. We apparently swallow air all day long, but little of the nitrogen in the atmosphere is present in the gas we pass each day. So it seems likely that most gas in swallowed air is eructated, not passed along. Some individuals may be unconsciously or consciously (if they are using esophageal speech after removal of the voice box) aspirating air into the esophagus and part of this may end up in the stomach. How much of the stomach air passes into the duodenum and the upper bowel may be influenced by posture, according to Levitt. Lying down in the supine position on our back makes eructation difficult because gas is trapped by liquid covering the esophageal junction with the stomach.

2. Carbon dioxide (CO_2) is released from the interaction of the acid (hydrogen ions) of the stomach with the bicarbonates (HCO_3) of the pancreas and duodenum. But this CO_2 is rapidly absorbed in the upper intestine and contributes little to rectal gas.

3. The major rectal gases are hydrogen (H_2), carbon dioxide (CO_2), and methane (CH_4), all of which are produced by colonic bacteria acting on the undigested complex carbohydrates and starches that reach the colon. When the small intestine is invaded by colonic bacteria, these gases are liberated into the small bowel as well. It should be remembered that these gases are odorless. The smell of flatus and stool is due to traces of other materials. Indoles and skatoles were assumed in the past to be responsible for the odor. Now it is felt that sulphur-containing compounds, such as methanethiol and dimethyl sulfide, are the culprits.

What Can Be Done about the Gas Problem?

Air-swallowing is essentially a functional tic and I have in the section on non-ulcer dyspepsia (Chapter 4) mentioned the variety of maneuvers that have been suggested to reduce air-swallowing: chewing rather than gulping food, eating and drinking slowly, and avoiding animated conversations during mealtimes.

Abdominal bloating and distention are probably not due to excessive gas—"too much" gas in the intestine—but rather is due to the ability of some foods to stimulate abnormal motility in the stomach or intestine, which seem related to the irritable bowel syndrome.

At present, alterations in the diet have been the basic approach of healthy individuals who suffer from these complaints, but good evidence is hard to come by. In persons who are lactose intolerant, reduction of milk product intake, the use of oral lactase enzyme preparations, such as Lactaid®, and substitutions of yogurt rather than milk, for example, has helped some individuals. An enzyme preparation (Beano®), an alpha-galactosidase, reduces gas by-products after eating a meal containing beans, and from time to time, activated charcoal is prescribed for gas reduction, but the evidence here is not terribly convincing. There is some anecdotal evidence that exercise helps with gas as well.

Excessive Rectal Gas

Almost all the patients treated by Dr. Levitt who complained of excessive gas produced hydrogen and methane in the colon.

The hydrogen and carbon dioxide may indicate fermentation of malabsorbed sugars due to a general abnormality of carbohydrate absorption or a more specific defect such as *lactase deficiency*. In these persons, a diet low in lactose (the sugar of milk), starches, or legumes will reduce gas formation, but these diets are tedious to follow and few individuals, unless plagued terribly, soon will not stick to the guidelines. After all, the "gassy" vegetables form an endless list—navy beans, soybeans, lima beans, onions, broccoli, cabbage, brussels sprouts, kohlrabi, radishes, cucumbers, and celery. And then there are the fruits that induce flatulence: apples, grapes and prune juice, raisins, and bananas, but curiously not orange juice or apricot nectar.

A Dietary Approach to Excessive Gas

The dietary approach to excessive gas attempts to reduce the amount of fermentable material that escapes intestinal absorption and thus contributes to the mixture on which the colon bacteria thrive. Again, studies of Dr. Michael Levitt are pertinent. When normal individuals are fed meals containing different complex carbohydrates—oats, whole wheat, potatoes, corn, and cooked beans—all reveal the interesting malabsorption of these carbohydrates, except for rice. So it seems that the fermentable, nonabsorbable material, even in normal individuals, is starch.

A legendary individual has been cited in the medical literature—a twenty-eight-year-old man studied by Dr. Levitt. This young man recorded each passage of rectal gas over a three-year period. He passed gas thirty-four times a day, while seven match-controlled individuals passed gas only fourteen times. Most of this patient's gas was hydrogen and carbon dioxide produced in the colon. By reducing his milk intake, he helped his problem a bit, since this patient was deficient in the enzyme lactase. While the volume of his gas decreased, it wasn't normalized when he avoided milk. By means of elimination diets, the patient developed a diet that decreased his gas—the successful diet was restricted in carbohydrates, particularly wheat products.

It is also interesting, as well as pertinent, that patients who complain of having too much gas when they are studied carefully by modern techniques do not have excessive amounts of gas, but seem to be more sensitive to the amounts they have. This would be consistent with listing flatulence as part of an irritable bowel syndrome.

So remember that passing some gas by rectum is perfectly normal and a physiological by-product of digestion. It is the excessive flatulence that troubles us. For twenty-five normal individuals on their regular diet, the average number of times they passed gas in twenty-four hours was 10 ± 1 times/day, the upper limit of normal (mean ± 250) was 20 times/day.

15
* * *

DIET AND
THE AGING GUT

In the United States, the fastest growing sector of the population is the 65-and-over age group, currently numbering about 28 million. Students of demographics project that by the year 2050 one out of every eight of us will be 75 years and older. We all experience the effects of age on our bodies and can see its visible mark, but what does time do to the gut?

While age does make a difference, on the whole, the structure and workings of the organs of the digestive system are relatively spared many of the dramatic effects of age, unlike the central nervous system and the cardiovascular organs.

Does the Passage of Time Influence the Functioning of the Gastrointestinal Tract?

The short answer to this question is yes, but to a very limited extent.

Let us run through the entire tract. The *mouth*, the taste buds of the tongue, tend to decline in number as well as in their sharpness of function. The *salivary glands* may atrophy a bit with aging and thus lose their ability to moisten our food, and may diminish our pleasure in tasting our meals. Swallowing does not become disturbed with age, but the swallowing mechanism can be upset by the illnesses of age: stroke, diabetes, Parkinson's disease, and the medicines used to treat parkinsonism. The *stomach* makes less acid, both when resting and when stimulated by our meals, but I don't think this causes much trouble. Yet the diminution in acids may lead to less antisepsis and sterilization of the upper gut leading to bacterial overgrowth. This may on occasion lead to diarrhea. The *pancreas* suffers no effects from aging. As we grow older, both men and women develop gallstones equally. And removal of these gallstones may lead to diarrhea, which is somehow related to the bile salts and a condition called *bile salt catharsis* in which bile in the colon then causes diarrhea. Overall, our *intestines* will function less effectively than they did in our youth and adulthood, failing to absorb some substances, such as vitamins B1, B12, D, A, and its precursor substance beta-carotene, as well as folic acid (the vitamin needed to build red blood cells and hemoglobin). Functioning of the *colon* often slows down, and constipation becomes a constant complaint, most often due to decreased fiber intake and total bodily inaction.

Many of us also lose weight despite a good appetite, a good diet, and the absence of any obvious diseases of the intestine or other parts of the body. Part of this is because the intestine does not function as effectively as it did in earlier years, and we consequently absorb less of our intestinal contents. In addition to the vitamins which may no longer be absorbed as well, fats, too, may fail to be absorbed, and there are hints that the sugars of a carbohydrate breakfast may be incompletely absorbed.

In view of the current intense interest in calcium—because of its role in preventing osteoporosis in women and its possible role in lowering high blood pressure and even in protecting against colonic cancer—you should know it does seem reasonably certain that calcium absorption declines with age. The reasons for this are complex and include the failure of intestinal cells to function optimally, and the problems of diminished vitamin D absorption which helps absorption of calcium. By contrast, iron seems to be absorbed reasonably well in the older age groups, as are most drugs.

The causes of these variations with age are not clearly known. The aging *liver* makes normal amounts of bile, and the aging pancreas in its protected interior of the body makes adequate amounts of the enzymes needed for fat and protein digestion, so they do not help explain the decreased efficiency of the aging gut. Instead, it is reasonable to believe that the cells of the intestine which absorb digested materials either are sparser as we age or do not function as effectively as they did earlier in life. It seems unlikely that the blood flow to the intestine is at fault, as some have claimed.

Changes in the *colonic bacteria* may also interfere with intestinal absorption as we age. These organisms may migrate upstream into the small bowel, causing so-called bacterial overgrowth, and share the host's diet and impair normal absorption—which results in diarrhea. Sometimes this symptom may result from the low acidity of the older stomach (acid normally acts as an antiseptic sterilizing agent) or disturbances in the "housekeeping" waves of motion, which normally sweep through the small intestine but now fail to sweep this bacterial overgrowth out of the aging upper bowel. Some older individuals who are malnourished and have diarrhea may have bacterial overgrowth without any apparent cause. Antibiotics may be a great help to these people but result in antibiotic-associated diarrhea in turn.

The Aging Colon

People often experience an increased difficulty in moving their bowels with age. A gradual decrease in the amount of stool passed becomes apparent around age 65. Some of this may be due to loss of teeth and the choice of a softer, less fibrous diet; diminished food intake (because it is boring to eat alone after the death of a spouse); and changes in the intestine's muscular activity in the very old, as well as diminished general muscular activity. This constipation may also be the result of neurological degeneration, or the cumulative effect of years of taking laxatives that were effective before, as well as the effects of parkinsonism or the drugs used to treat parkinsonism.

General Aspects of Nutrition in the Older Age Groups

There is no evidence that any food or supplements (vitamins) can retard the aging process of the gastrointestinal tract. But it is important that we continue to eat a healthy diet and do not develop any serious deficiencies because we are eating less of our usual diet. The intake of calcium and iron-containing foods must be carefully continued.

There is no evidence that the aging gut needs a special diet of bland foods. If anything, quite the contrary. Since your taste buds and salivary glands aren't behaving as they once did, you may want to use your kitchen spices a bit more liberally. And you will want to make certain that grain and fiber are still a part of every meal. If we wish to prevent or correct the constipation that seems to accompany the aging process, low-impact exercise, such as walking briskly, will also tone up all our muscles, including abdominal and intestinal muscles needed for bowel evacuation. Whatever program of diet and general lifestyle has kept you well until the category of old age, whether the "young" old of 65 to 80, or the "old" old of 80 and above, stick with it. Do not fall into the trap of food fads.

If your teeth are giving you trouble, then correct your teeth. Don't skip meals because it is boring to prepare them or because you don't enjoy eating them. Your gut needs fiber in adequate amounts to prevent constipation and to maintain your health. Aging is not a sickness!

Specific Nutrition in the Aged

Recent studies have indicated that perhaps 70 percent of the population 70 years and older do have some degree of difficulty absorbing some substances of their dietary intake and the possible effects of this are under study. This problem of absorption is not the result of heart disease or blood flow through the intestines. As a result, many older persons should take supplements with certain minerals and vitamins. *Folic acid*, or folate, is one of the substances that older people lack; it is found in green leafy vegetables, liver, wheat germ, dried peas, and beans. *Vitamin B6* is also deficient in some older individuals and can be obtained from whole wheat bread, cereal, liver, avocados, spinach, green beans, bananas, and fish. A considerable fuss has been made over vitamin B12 deficiency which, it is suggested, causes memory loss, disorientation, balance and coordination problems. These symptoms may result from a condition known as *atrophic gastritis* that commonly occurs in 60- to 80-year-olds. In this condition, the stomach's secretions diminish, and this may explain the inability to absorb vitamin B12 from foods. Folic acid and B12 can be absorbed in tablet form and are contained in most multivitamins.

Problems with *calcium* can contribute to osteoporosis, with the loss of bone and minerals, and may lead to fractures. A number of factors are believed to play a contributing role: high-protein diets, smoking, or sedentary lifestyle, coupled with a low intake of calcium in the diet, which is presumed to be the most important factor. The difference of opinion on the needed daily requirements of calcium has been discussed in Chapter 3. The typical American woman appears to take only about half of the recommended daily amount of calcium, which is currently 1500 milligrams. The most popular calcium supplement, calcium carbonate, present in Tums®, is not well absorbed. The best sources are dairy foods like milk and yogurt. Be sure to look for the low-fat and nonfat forms. Foods rich in calcium include collard greens, peas, broccoli, canned salmon, and sardines because of the small bones. But the proper absorption of calcium is dependent on vitamin D which is often underconsumed. Milk is fortified with vitamin D, and fatty fish like mackerel, salmon, and sardines are rich sources as well.

I have already mentioned the antioxidants in Chapter 3. These include vitamins C and E, as well as beta-carotene, which is converted into vitamin A. Diets rich in vitamin C and beta-carotene seem to protect people against heart attacks, lower the blood pressure, and lower the incidence of several cancers. Although the complete story is not available, the apparent safety of large doses of vitamin E has prompted many experts to recommend daily supplements in the range of 200 to 400 International Units (IUs), especially after the age of 50. It is not possible to consume enough vitamin E from our foods without adding a great deal of fat. There is less agreement about vitamin C because megadoses cause problems like diarrhea and kidney stones and may interfere with the absorption of vitamin B12. There is no agreement on beta-carotene as a supplement.

So my advice is simple: eat plenty of food rich in carotenoids—carrots, dark green vegetables like spinach and broccoli, cantaloupe, and sweet potatoes.

16

❋ ❋ ❋

CAN DIET *MAKE*
A DIFFERENCE?

What we eat can and does affect our health. Investigations into the relationship of nutrition and human disease have a long-standing history stretching back to Lind, who discovered that lime juice could prevent and cure scurvy, and even before. But it is in the twentieth century that nutrition came of age and its biochemical pathways became science. It is the vitamin C in lime juice that is important, and we are just beginning to isolate other substances in our diet that can help us combat other diseases.

Diet plays an important role in a considerable number of medical disorders and it is what is missing, as well as what is present, that plays a part. It is common knowledge that overeating leads to *obesity* with the added risks of heart disease and diabetes. But there is clear evidence that components missing from the diet can also cause specific medical conditions. Congenital lack of a digestive enzyme may lead to phenylketonuria with brain damage in the newborn. Inadequate folic acid in the diet of a pregnant woman will lead to structural damage in the infant's brain and spinal cord. Hence diet is an essential concern of both patients and physicians in treating and preventing many general medical disorders.

The primary concern of this book is the role of diet in preventing and treating disorders of the gastrointestinal tract and its related digestive glands—the liver, gallbladder, and pancreas.

Our instinct tells us that what we eat should play some part in the health of our digestive system, but if you have read this book carefully, you already know there are large gaps in our information that still remain to be filled in, and so I have put the title of this final chapter in the form of a question: Can Diet *Make* a Difference?—not only because the gaps remain, but because almost each day the newspaper reports revisions and updates of yesterday's solid facts. Margarine was O.K. for a long time but now should be eliminated from our diet because it contains the *trans* forms of fat rather than the safe *cis* form.

I have been a gastroenterologist for a great many patients over a long time and I have attempted to distill what I have learned from this experience knowing full well that what we think is solid today may change with the onslaught of newer nutritional information.

In Part I of this book, which deals essentially with eating for health, I tackle the very difficult question of whether the ideal diet exists. Despite continuing controversies by the authorities and researchers in the field, there is at present at least the beginning of a consensus.

We must consume enough calories to maintain the healthy structure and workings of the human machine and the output of energy needed for all the tasks we ask this intricate machine to accomplish. *But* we must avoid, if possible, getting overweight. Obesity carries risks for coronary heart disease, hereditary diabetes, elevated blood pressure, and even some tumors (ovary and colon). Yet we are learning every day that the control of food intake in humans and in animals is under the influence of complex chemical messengers (hormones) and receptive centers in the mid-brain. We no longer scold the overweight.

Here is a list of guidelines all of us should adopt in our diets:

- We must reduce our intake of fat. Most Americans get 40 percent of their daily calories from fat, and this should be dramatically reduced to at least 30 percent and, if possible, even lower.
- We need especially to reduce the fat derived from animal and dairy products: substituting the polyunsaturated fats of olive and corn oils for the saturated fats of palm oil and coconut oil, which many of the cooking and frying fats contain. An egg yolk contains 300 milligrams of cholesterol and should be restricted, especially if your cholesterol is high.
- We must increase the number of daily portions of vegetables, grains, and salads, for their fiber content, low-fat content, high-vitamin content, and some as yet unidentified elements that protect against cancer. We must consume at least 5 to 8 servings of this food group each day.
- We should aim for a daily intake of 30 to 40 grams of fiber— a diet suitable for a digestive track that evolved in the Paleolithic Age.
- Women must take larger doses of calcium, up to 1500 milligrams daily, along with vitamin D, to prevent osteoporosis. And pregnant women must take adequate amounts of folic acid to ensure the health of their newborns.
- It seems prudent, at least at present, to take a supplement containing the antioxidants: vitamin C, beta-carotene (the precursor of vitamin A), and vitamin E (alpha tocopherol).
- With a normal diet, protein intake will take care of itself and the needs for trace elements (zinc and selenium) will be satisfied.

If we can maintain this type of diet, we are close to the diet our Paleolithic ancestors lived on. In this way we may avoid the difficulties that have arisen from the fact that our inherited intestinal tract may not be prepared to handle the enormously changed and prepared foods of today.

We have systematically proceeded down the alimentary tract to consider the role of diet in preventing, causing, and treating gastrointestinal disorders. Diet plays a definite but limited role most of the time, with several major exceptions.

- Celiac disease (sprue) is caused by a reaction to the protein gluten of wheat, rice, oats, and barley and responds dramatically to the withdrawal of gluten from the diet.
- Oxalate kidney stones in inflammatory bowel disease (ulcerative colitis and Crohn's disease) require a low-oxalate diet along with other precautions.

The treatment of several diseases includes diet as an integral part. Let me highlight what we have learned.

- For *all* digestive disorders, cigarette smoking, alcohol, and caffeine must be avoided.
- The ulcer group (esophagitis, gastritis, gastric and duodenal ulcer) responds better to current therapies where the diet is bland, low in acidity, and regularly spaced.
- Gallstones—basically a metabolic disorder of the liver and its ability to form bile salts and cholesterol, in which bile stagnates in the gallbladder—seem less likely to form if we maintain a low-fat diet and regularly spaced meals. These changes in diet may also prevent severe attacks of biliary colic.
- Pancreatitis requires complete cessation of alcohol and a low-fat diet when it is precipitated by alcohol or that form related to gallbladder disease.
- The irritable bowel syndrome (digestive complaints without an organic basis) is difficult to treat dietetically, but some individuals do better with the avoidance of irritants, food intolerances, and allergies discovered either by chance or on elimination diets.
- Constipation in the form not associated with organic disease requires a high-fiber diet daily.

- A high-fiber diet is essential in preventing the development of colonic, especially sigmoid, diverticula and diverticulitis.
- Unfortunately, for the inflammatory bowel diseases (ulcerative colitis and Crohn's disease), we know little regarding the role of diet in causing these disorders. Here a well-balanced, high caloric, somewhat lower fiber intake dietary program seems reasonable.
- For cancer of the colon and rectum, a low-fat and high-fiber diet is important in preventing these cancers, along with generous portions of fruit, vegetables, and salad.
- Intestinal gas is difficult to treat. For some individuals, a high-fiber diet with some reduction of complex carbohydrates (vegetables and starches) may help.

The aging gut does rather well as time goes by in contrast to the cardiac and central nervous systems. One must not let weariness, loneliness, bad teeth, or apathy interfere with the continuation of a well-balanced, normal diet which this book has stressed.

Appendix
✹ ✹ ✹

DRUGS AND NUTRITION

Calcium Absorption

With all the current focus on osteoporosis and the many factors which may influence its development (lack of exercise, cigarette smoking, decline in estrogen in women after menopause), a great deal of attention has been paid to the question of getting enough calcium into our system from our foods. Now attention is being paid to medications that may interfere with the absorption of calcium or adversely affect the bone density of certain bone cells, especially the bone-building cells. Cortisone derivatives, the so-called glucocorticoid list of drugs, are synthetic versions of the steroids produced by the human adrenal gland and are widely used in diseases like arthritis, asthma, allergy, inflammatory bowel disease (both Crohn's and ulcerative colitis), forms of cancer and lupus, as well as in transplantations. These drugs can lead to difficulties with calcium absorption and can rapidly cause bone loss. They also increase the loss of calcium from the kidney. (These valuable but potent drugs include cortisone, hydrocortisone, prednisone, prednisolone, and methylprednisolone, among others.)

Several other drugs have been found to affect calcium in the body. Thyroid hormone, widely prescribed in the United States for patients deficient in thyroid activity under the trade name of Synthroid®, can cause bone loss. Phenytoin (Dilantin®), an antiseizure drug, has also been found to cause bone loss.

It is also suggested that large amounts of aluminum-containing antacids can influence the calcium in our bones, weakening them especially in individuals with poor kidney function. Maalox®, Rolaids®, Gelusil®, and Gaviscon® all contain aluminum. Other over-the-counter aids like Tums®, which do not contain aluminum, may be substituted.

Care must be exercised with the drug *cholestyramine* (Questran®), which is used to lower blood cholesterol levels. This compound, too, may influence calcium absorption indirectly.

Methotrexate, used for several conditions—cancer, immune disorders, arthritis (especially the psoriatic form)—has toxic effects on the cells that form new bone and can lead to disruption of kidney function with increased loss of calcium in the urine.

Cyclosporine, used to suppress rejection of transplants, has been found to lead to bone loss.

And the gonadotropin-releasing hormone analogs, used to treat endometriosis, have been associated with bone loss, especially in those women who start off with a low bone mass to begin with.

Considering all these drugs and their widespread use, it is not surprising that many physicians recommend a daily supplement of calcium, especially for women over fifty. I would agree with this recommendation and suggest 1500 milligrams of calcium daily.

Table 13. Influence of Food on Drug Absorption

Food Impairs Absorption of	*Food Enhances Absorption of*
Many antibiotics	Propanolol
Aspirin	Hydralazine
Propatheline	Hydrochlorothiazide
L-dopa	Propoxyphene
Methyldopa	Griseofulvin
Rifampin	Nitrofurantoin
Isoniazid	Spironolactone
Phenobarbital	
Methotrexate	
Acetaminophen	
Digoxin	
Furosemide	
Potassium ions	

Food on the other hand may alter the absorption of medications, at times imparing their absorption, at other times increasing their absorption.

It is important to remember also that drugs can influence the absorption of other medicines, vitamins, and nutrients as seen in Table 14 on the following page.

Table 14. Drugs That Can Influence the Absorption of Other Medicines, Vitamins, and Nutrients

Drug or Type	May Affect Absorption of
Antacids	Tetracycline
antacids containing aluminum	Diazepam
or magnesium in regular doses	Cimetidine
antacids in large doses	Nitrofurantoin
	Penicillin G
	Sulfa drugs
	Isoniazid
	Digoxin
	Phenytoin
	Chlorpromazine
	Propanolol
Antibiotics	
Tetracycline	Iron
Sulfasalazine	Folic acid
Antimetabolites	
Colchicine	Folic acid
	Vitamin B12
Anticonvulsants	
Phenytoin	Folic acid
Oral contraceptives	Folic acid
Cholestyramine	Aspirin, chlorothiazide
	Iron, phenobarbital

LOW-FAT COOKBOOKS
✻ ✻ ✻

In the Kitchen with Rosie: Oprah's Favorite Recipes (Knopf, $14.95) by Rosie Daly. A favorite at present and a best seller that contains reasonable advice on the use of evaporated skim milk, nonfat cottage cheese, nonfat mayonnaise, and nonfat yogurt.

The Mediterranean Diet Cookbook (Bantam, $27.95) by Nancy Harmon. This is a reasonable presentation of the Mediterranean pyramid—low in saturated fat—with sound advice on olive oil, a monounsaturated fat.

Provencal Light (Bantam $29.95) by Martha Rose Shulman. This book advocates low-fat cooking, but avoids extremes.

The Wellness Low-Fat Cookbook (Rebus/Random House, $24.95) from the University of California at Berkeley. This is considered one of the most scientific, sound contributions to the low-fat movement.

SUBJECT INDEX

✳ ✳ ✳